WITS|GUTS|GRIT

WITS | GUTS | GRIT

All-Natural Biohacks for Raising Smart, Resilient Kids

Jena Pincott

CHICAGO
REVIEW
PRESS

Library of Congress Cataloging-in-Publication Data

Names: Pincott, J. (Jena), author.
Title: Wits guts grit : all-natural biohacks for raising smart, resilient
    kids / Jena Pincott.
Description: First edition. | Chicago, Illinois : Chicago Review Press,
    [2018] | Includes bibliographical references and index.
Identifiers: LCCN 2017040060 (print) | LCCN 2017045617 (ebook) | ISBN
    9781613736890 (adobe pdf) | ISBN 9781613736913 (epub) | ISBN
    9781613736906 (kindle) | ISBN 9781613736883 (trade paper)
Subjects: LCSH: Child rearing. | Resilience (Personality trait) in children.
    | Gifted children. | BISAC: FAMILY & RELATIONSHIPS / Parenting /
    General. | MEDICAL / Immunology.
Classification: LCC HQ769 (ebook) | LCC HQ769 .P6625 2018 (print) |
    DDC 649/.1—dc23
LC record available at https://lccn.loc.gov/2017040060

Cover design: Andrew Brozyna
Cover images: Blueberries, hands, moon, bacteria, and gardening,
    iStockPhoto.com; feet, Shutterstock.
Typesetting: Nord Compo

Printed in the United States of America
5 4 3 2 1

To Una Joy, whose curiosity and love of nature inspire me,
and to Amandine, my next guinea pig

Contents

Introduction

WHEN IT COMES to raising smart and resilient kids, there's nature and there's nurture. This book looks at natural "biohacks" that help kids adapt to a challenging and continuously changing world, so it involves a little bit of nature (genes and instinct) and a lot of nurture (environment, upbringing, and interventions). How much sway nurture has over nature is a mystery that even my six-year-old, "UJ," touched on the other night when she asked, "Mama, if we went back to the wild, would we become like our ancient ancestors again?" She basically wanted to know if we'd be better people if we left our trappings and lived and ate like our forebears in a more natural setting. I should mention that this was coming from a city kid who has never spent a night outdoors or even seen a real campfire. Here, in New York City, the wild animals are rats.

"Hmmm," I said with suspicion, looking at the clock on her nightstand: 8:24. A deep question like this struck me as a ploy to stay up late on a school night. "Depends on what you mean by natural. It's hard to tell with humans."

This was a deeply unsatisfactory response, especially because I punctuated it with darkness, turning off her light and promising her a better answer at a better time. But after I kissed her good night, the question lingered.

Before becoming a parent, I never gave much thought to the nature-nurture dynamic—the interplay of innate qualities versus learned or acquired ones. I was more focused on futurism, the next big thing. Then UJ arrived, followed four and a half years later by her sister, Ami. There were primal smells in the air: blood, milk, feces, sweat, tears. It occurred to me that for these two young mammals to survive and thrive in the world, they'd need wits, guts, and a lot of grit. What is it, I wondered, that shapes kids' temperament, personality, brainpower, emotional resilience, self-regulation, memory, powers of focus, mental flexibility, and the plasticity of their neurons? I had a suspicion that outside forces I'm not aware of, and over which I have no control, could have as much impact on these virtues as any play-group, extracurricular, or reading list I'd foist upon them. I've never so much wanted to have control, and I'd never been so desperate to cede it to a higher power.

Ultimately, it all comes down to the interaction of biology and environment. I first started to think about invisible forces (the "nature" or "biology" side of the equation) when UJ was a colicky, sensitive infant. Many people told me that what you see is what you get; that temperament is basically set by age two. Around this same time, microbiome research busted out—first in geeky science circles, then later in the mainstream. The field, which focuses on the impact of gut bacteria on human health and development, has grown even faster than my kids. Now we know that some microbes within the gut release signaling molecules, such as neurotransmitters serotonin and dopamine, that modulate our moods and behavior. There's increasing evidence that specific types of bacteria contribute to the ability to bounce back after a setback. Recently, a study on the brain-gut link found a striking correlation between toddler temperament and gut bacteria, with a diversity of microbes associated with extraversion and certain strains with introversion.

Could the right gut bacteria dial up my own kids' resilience and grittiness or somehow optimize their temperament and even their brain development? I wondered. If so, how do we get some (the "nurture" side of the equation)?

This is where "biohacking" comes in. I use the loose definition of "biohack": to use self-experimentation to explore and tinker with body, mind, and biology to help reach your full potential (or, in this case, your kids' potential). (If you saw the word *biohack* in the title and thought this was an illicit guide for programming your child to be a Teflon genius, I'm sorry to disappoint.) Experimentation here is low-tech and cheap, mostly using natural resources that we all have or that are acquired easily. The aim is to explore subtle but effective ways to support joy, learning, creativity, and, most of all, resilience in our children.

Because the pressure's on! My grade-schooler, like many kids, hardly stepped out of the sandbox and is already knee-deep in expectations: music performances, school plays, word problems, and critical thinking. In her future, there will be grades and standardized tests, then high school and college placement. There will be performance pressure, both social and academic. There will be perils and pitfalls, some of which are experienced by every generation and, I worry, some unique to hers. My kid knows that the adults in her life expect (OK, hope) that she'll pull herself up by her bootstraps and rebound.

We all want to see *grit*—a term popularized by the psychologist Angela Duckworth that describes the ability to keep pursuing something even after setbacks and sometimes against all odds. Gritty kids know and accept that mistakes and failings are part of learning, and they get comfortable with the feeling of struggle. They bounce back. Resilience leads to better health, happiness, and success in life. The good news is that children are not born with a set amount of resilience. It's a muscle that we can help them strengthen. What a gift it would be to learn "gritty" resilience-building behaviors while still young, so that they become habit.

We're accustomed to thinking of grit as a mindset. But as parents and educators, we often overlook the factors that underlie grit or are "ingredients" of grit or grit-related virtues like focus, trust, cognitive flexibility, working memory, stamina, and ability to self-regulate and cope with anxiety. To this list I include several items that, in turn, underlie these qualities: missing microbes and micronutrients; bodily awareness, physical contact, and physicality; light, air, a stronger connection with our environment (including ways to overcome challenges of living in adverse settings like cities); and even oddball stuff like the biological signals in sweat and tears. What if we tap into those forces?

This book was conceived by *what-if* questions, and those questions inspired explorations and experiments. Starting with microbes, I wondered *what if* we identify the ones that support stress resilience, find ways to expose ourselves to them, and then test ourselves? Moving on to micronutrients, I wondered: *What if* we reintroduce a mineral that's deficient in almost every child's diet; would it reduce anxiety and increase bounce back, as the science now suggests? *What if* memory and learning could improve measurably after eating certain foods high in plant chemicals called flavonols? *What if* we reintroduce nature to our lives; will it help modern problems like attention deficit and mind wandering? *What if* we bring darkness back into the evening, the way it used to be, or tinker with the school and house lights: how would that affect thinking? *What if* kids could be trained to tune in to their own biology—from racing hearts and lurching stomachs to breathing patterns and sweat signals—and use those bodily cues to ace a performance? *What if* primal ways of moving the body strengthen kids' working memory or put them in a more limber mindset? *What if* receiving the right types of touch can translate into better emotional control and self-regulation? Doctors and psychologists rarely address these types of questions.

Each month I looked at a new topic or question, often involving a form of experiment or "biohack," drawing on peer-reviewed studies in microbiology, neuroscience, cognitive science, psychology, nutrition, behavioral epigenetics, and other fields. In some cases, my family tried to stage an experiment to replicate those that took place in the lab. I provide information in the chapters for how you, the reader, can experiment with your own children too. My personal experiences described here are for fun and exploration and are not meant to be comprehensive or draw conclusions. As the primatologist Irwin Bernstein once said, "The plural of anecdote is not data." These are anecdotes. If there ever are antidotes, they're in the scientific papers described. (Bear in mind, however, that the science is always unfolding and further research is always warranted before conclusions can be drawn. What works for my family might not work for yours. The theme here is experimentation.)

Don't force yourself to read this book chronologically if you're otherwise inclined. Dip in anywhere that interests you. Some of the findings are new and surprising; others draw on older wisdom on which I attempt to shed new light. Because this is a book about children, I always looked for and prioritized pediatric research, but some studies were conducted only on adult subjects (and a few only on nonhumans). On the upside, almost all the findings here will benefit parents, too.

Beyond the desire to help our children be the best versions of themselves, this book is inspired by the idea of restoring nature, or some approximation of it, to childhood. The statistics here are galvanizing. Kids today spend less time in nature than any generation in the past. A poll taken by the Nature Conservancy found that only one in three American kids is physically active every day, and only 6 percent of middle-grade students play outside on their own. How is this generation going to protect and care for the natural environment if they're so distanced from it, both physically and psychologically?

Many of the investigations here touch on the ills that come of this "de-naturing" of childhood: too few microbes and minerals, too much air, light, and noise pollution (especially for city kids), and, often, too much of a disconnect from their own bodies and biological processes. This book attempts to home in on the deep connection between the microscopic, remote worlds of microbes, nutrients, hormones, neurons, and the like with the everyday realities of our kids' lives: friends, fears, risks, competition, growing pains, pressure, and play. It begins with microbes and ends with macros, a big picture of mental health and resilience.

As a science writer, I care about precision, considering how the science is often ambiguous or imperfect, in need of further investigation, and always contingent on new discoveries. As a parent, I like actionable, hands-on results (even when the science is preliminary). The tweaks and changes in this book have helped my family, of this I am sure. But even at their best, I think of these "biohacks"—with microbes, plant chemicals, mind, touch, and movement exercises, light experiments, and biofeedback—as little nudges rather than agents of dramatic change. They build on momentum that's already there.

The experiments herein may nudge children toward better bounce back from stressors, easier self-regulation, stickier memory, smoother interactions, sounder sleep, more satisfying performances, and stronger self-insight. All these tiny, optimizing efforts enrich and build on well-established grit-building techniques: to cultivate optimism and passion; to remember that failure and frustration are OK, even necessary, and fleeting; to step outside one's comfort zone; and to believe, truly, that we're always growing and evolving and never stuck. But a gritty mindset requires all the undergirding it can get; improving ourselves isn't always, well, instinctive.

Nor is parenting, for that matter. Parenting instinct, I believe, is as reliable as the "go back to nature" instinct. (Even the commonsense stuff, like physical affection, isn't as instinctive as you'd think.) If I were to give UJ a more thoughtful response to her bedtime question about whether humans could "rewild," I'd say it sure wouldn't come naturally. But we can use science to put us back in touch with nature and our biology in ways that help us most. We just need to explore and tinker, recover and discover. Which, come to think of it, sounds a lot like childhood itself.

I

Invisible Forces

JANUARY

Does Grit Depend on Guts?

---

*The good-guy microbes you want to hack
your kid's nervous system*

L AST SPRING, IN a monkey-themed bathroom in New York City, a mother and her four-year-old daughter undertook a science experiment. The girl, undies at her ankles, held a two-pronged Q-tip to a wad of used toilet paper. The mother controlled the child's wrist tensely. Together, they dabbed the swab in the brown matter.

"Great! Now we'll label this and send it to the lab," said the mom devoutly as she sealed the sample. "Scientists will test it. Then we'll know which types of bacteria live inside you!"

"No way, never in the *universe*," said the girl, my daughter, whose nickname is UJ. "My *name* on my *poop*?"

Is it just preschoolers, or do most people think that fecal bacteria are disgusting? Me, I proudly joined the counterculture and sent the (code-labeled) poop to American Gut, an open-source "citizen scientist" initiative that sequences and compares the microbiota of people everywhere in the country. The lab uses genetic sequencing technology that identifies gut bacteria by their DNA. In about a month we found out which microbes were in the guts of UJ and her infant sister, Ami, whose sample was acquired from her diaper without protest.

As believers in, well, the *movement*, you start hearing catchy slogans about the relationship between humans and their microbiome: *You're more microbe than mammal.* It's true; about half the cells in us are not human. There are trillions of bacteria that live within us and on us; we each have five hundred to one thousand species in the gut. *You're just a vessel for microbes.* The belly button alone harbors hundreds of species.

All the fervor and literal naval gazing has gained momentum in the past few years, and it's easy to understand why. A fast-growing body of research suggests that the trillions of microbial inhabitants that live within us have a deep, complex connection with our health and nervous systems—including our propensity for asthma, allergies, diabetes, and cancer—and, more mysteriously, with our brains and behavior. The bacteria that grow within a child's guts in the formative years may well have long-term, even lifelong consequences. Developmental pathways, influenced by bacteria, can become destiny. Everyone who follows this science is trying to find answers to the essential question: How do these inhabitants affect our growth, health, and behavior? Microbes may play a role in the ultimate mystery: *Why are we the way we are? And who are we anyway?*

The answer depends on the follow-up question: Who are *they*? So, during the long wait for the results that would list all the species in my kids' guts, I found myself surprisingly anxious. We had not prepped for this test. I flashed on UJ's veggie-light diet and my sugar addiction during both pregnancies. I'm a worrier, which is a quality I'd like my daughters to inherit only in moderation. The results, I consoled myself, would inspire us to make lifestyle changes going forward. The *before* profile, ugly as it might be, would make the *after* look even better.

There are many, many microbes within us, and their influence on health and mental health is immeasurable. For our purposes, it seemed appropriate to focus first on the types that are well studied and the most relevant to us. The ones associated with stress resilience.

Now, what the heck was on that Q-tip?

It's very clear that bacteria have been here much longer than we have, and as far as they're concerned, we may be just a passing feature in their history. —Stuart Levy

I'd been wanting to hack my kids with "stress-resilience" microbes ever since I heard about the discoveries in Ireland. Several years ago, at the University of Cork, a neuroscientist named John Cryan designed a simple experiment. Every day, he fed some of his lab mice a special broth that contained *Lactobacillus rhamnosus*. *Lactobacillus* is a genus of microbe that is common in some yogurt, and the dose of *L. rhamnosus* he gave them was, by human standards, about the same you might eat in a half cup of yogurt. No one expected the mice to get sick, and they didn't. In fact, not much seemed to happen.

Then, after several weeks, it was time for the mice to have a "forced swim," which is a gold-standard test for measuring endurance and resilience—in rodents, at least. It's a test that wouldn't be ethical if human children were made to do it. A mouse is dunked into a tall Plexiglas cylinder of water and left alone to struggle for six minutes. It's a bleak situation: the sudden immersion is shocking, the paddling is grueling, and the mouse doesn't know if it's ever going to end. Resilience is measured in the number of minutes the creature continues to tread water. Despair is measured in the amount of time it floats despondently. I found myself wondering what my kid would do.

To the surprise of all, the mice that were the likeliest to stay aloft, still kicking to the six-minute mark, were the ones fed the *Lactobacillus*. It's hard to tell with mice, but you might say they were less anxious and depressed by the situation than those that hadn't received the bacterial boost. They certainly had more fight and feistiness in the face of adversity. They were calmer, too: they produced only half the level of the stress hormone corticosterone as the control mice in the trial. You might even say they had more *grit*—that catchy catchall word that sums up perseverance and conscientiousness.

Around the same time, word had spread about gut bugs in the genus *Bifidobacterium* that seemed to have as soothing an effect on the nervous system as *L. rhamnosus*. Like lactobacilli, bifidobacteria, or Bifs for short, are common microbes in babies and have had a long, mutually satisfying relationship with their human hosts. We've been eating them in yogurt and sauerkraut and kimchi and other fermented foods for thousands of years.

If *Bifidobacterium* could make mice as gritty and calm in the face of adversity as *Lactobacillus* did, Cryan wanted the result to be clear and convincing. So for this study he used a strain of mice that are high-strung neurotics by nature. For six weeks, he fed them food that was enriched with one of two species of Bifs: *B. longum* (1714) or *B. breve* (1205), which are like cousins to each other. For a point of comparison, he also included two other groups of mice that either took an antidepressant, Lexapro, or ate a normal diet. Then he put them through the gauntlet: six minutes of the sink-or-swim test, six minutes of tail suspension, and exposure to an elevated maze in an open field (every instinct tells rodents they'll surely be raptor food if they don't find cover quickly, so this test is immensely stressful). Would the Bifs-fed mice bounce back better than the others?

There were telltale signs of a behavioral shift. First off, the treated mice were calmer in their cages. Stressed mice have a weird reflex to bury marbles obsessively, and there were fewer marbles at the bottom of the nests of *Bifidobacterium-* or Lexapro-fed mice. While all three groups despaired during the forced swim test (unlike the *L. rhamnosus*–fed mice), the Bifs-fed subjects excelled in other tests of stamina. Mice usually freeze up when hung by their tails, but the *B. longum* mice were 40 percent more resilient, fighting with their hearts in their mouths to free themselves from their predicament even as their peers went limp. In the elevated maze with open air, the control mice and those fed Lexapro panicked while those treated with *B. breve* were more persistent and exploratory. *Braver.*

Stamina is one part of resilience, or grit. Bravery is another. You might say that the ability to learn under pressure is a third. How well do any of us learn under stress? The lucky ones, like my husband, seem to thrive on it. Others, like me, may despair and stop learning or doing their best work, and the underlying nervous system has a lot to do with which camp you're in. Could *Bifidobacterium* also help animals retain new information under stress? Not a bad skill for a child to have in a high-pressure world.

Again, Cryan recruited a breed of innately nervous mice and fed them Bifs for eleven weeks. This time, however, instead of testing for resilience, he tested them for cognitive abilities. How well could they discriminate between two objects? How efficiently could they navigate a maze, learning from their wrong turns and dead ends and not making the same mistakes twice? Even on a symbolic level, an improvement here would be a victory. And indeed, to the delight of geeky enthusiasts who were following Cryan's work closely, myself included, the mice with the Bifs boost had lower error rates and faster runs. Think for second about what it takes to achieve this: a calmness of mind, an ability to be present in the moment, a stronger memory, and the stamina to make mistakes and not get discouraged.

Many tests of a psychoactive substance start like this, with animal research. But it's somewhat of an anthropomorphic leap to assume that the forced swim test or the buried marble test predicts human resilience. So when enough successes have been achieved, studies on people begin.

By now, Cryan was ready to move from rodents to men, which wasn't a risky leap. Bifidobacteria are harmless bacteria, and while *B. longum* isn't available in many brands of supermarket yogurt in the United States, it's not so exotic that you can't find it if you look hard enough. So, for four weeks daily, he gave a group of male volunteers a serving of yogurt with either *B. longum* or a cultured-yogurt-like placebo. Every day, the men answered questions about life's big and little stresses. *Do you feel like things are going your way? How often today have you been upset because of something that happened unexpectedly?*

Somewhere between weeks three and four, the end of the month-long experiment, it became apparent that the men's daily stress level was lower in the *B. longum* group than in the placebo group, as were their cortisol levels when they took a cold stressor test (immersing one's hands in freezing water under vaguely hostile observation). When Cryan's team tested the men's memory, the *B. longum*–fed group showed subtle enhancements compared to controls. What made these results so captivating is that the volunteers didn't know whether the yogurt they were eating contained *B. longum* or not. It was a blind study.

Fall seven times, stand up eight. —Japanese Proverb

For a four-year-old, violin practice can be like a forced swim. Even a six-minute session can feel like forever—for daughter and mother both—and UJ didn't have a sense of when or how, or if, it would ever end. "Bow evenly," I'd implore. "Scroll up! Curvy rainbow pinkie!" Sink or swim! A typical session might involve playing rhythms in a sequence. Halfway through, without fail, the child would sink to the floor. There, she'd obsess about a microscopic scratch on her finger or demand Indian food.

There are reasons why things weren't working out in the beginning. My preschooler wasn't necessarily ready to play an instrument. Mama was too critical. I was heavily pregnant with Ami, and my fatigue and irritability didn't help. UJ's negative mood was compounded by colds; wave after wave of them, they'd dull and crush her.

"May I whisper something in your ear?" she'd ask.

"Yes."

"You don't love me," she'd hiss.

"Prove it," I'd say, as lightly I could. This was my standard response.

Again, she'd sink to the floor and go belly-up. In the psych lab, this would be called tanking.

Although violin practice is not as bad now, a year later, there are still sessions with tensions. It also isn't the only stress in her young life. There's always something. This year an older, oversized girl at school won't let anyone else pretend to be kittens unless they follow her fickle rules. That's stressful. Learning new stuff is fun but stressful: computing super bonds and Sudoku grids, and making sure a lowercase *p* dangles below the bottom line rather than sitting on top of it. Sustained attention in the classroom is stressful, and the day is long. There are many, many ways in which resilience is tested and taxed in a child's day.

Everyone agrees that success in life requires "grit," a mix of resilience, tenacity, and determination. The psychologist Angela Duckworth, who put grit on the parental radar, names it as one of the two traits that predict achievement (the other is self-control). Grit, she found, is more predictive of success than IQ. A gritty kid isn't discouraged by setbacks, or at least not discouraged enough to set her back for long. She sees the big picture. She doesn't lose interest in something easily, and she works hard. She has stamina.

Many factors, of course, contribute to grit in the way the term has been popularized. Kids need to be praised for their effort. They need to learn the value of struggle. They must learn how to fail, and they gain resilience from repeated experiences in recovering after failure. They learn when they see parents and role models struggle and succeed. They learn by adapting.

But there's a factor, often overlooked, that all too often gums up grit: anxiety. If your stress response is a knee-jerk flare-up, it's hard to be resilient and focused. When I get down on the floor with UJ and hug her when she's despairing, I can feel her heart beating like a trapped dove. The first step in gaining resilience, it seems, is to tamp down the stress response that undermines it. Could bifidobacteria and lactobacillus help?

I learned a lesson I'd never forget. The lesson was that, when you have setbacks and failures, you can't overreact to them. —Angela Duckworth

UJ did not forget that her poop had been sent to a lab. For weeks, she asked me if the results were in. I remember hearing myself swallow when they finally arrived, via an e-mail link. Of the sixty or so genera listed on the report, I immediately ran my finger down to *Bifidobacterium* and *Lactobacillus*. UJ's *Bifidobacterium* represented about 3 percent of her gut microbiome, and her *Lactobacillus* hovered around 1 percent. Normal. The amount of *Bifidobacterium* in the gut is usually 5 percent or less in American kids, whether they were breast-fed or formula-fed early in life.

Of the species of Bifs in UJ's gut, however, there was no trace of *B. breve* or *B. longum*, the stars of Cryan's experiments. Of the *Lactobacillus*, there was no *L. rhamnosus*. (The current sequencing tests available to the public provide raw data for percentage of species such as *B. longum* in a specimen but unfortunately don't drill down to subspecies such as *B. longum* spp. *infantis* or strains such as *B. longum 1714*.)

Going by percentages of lactobacilli and bifidobacteria, the clear winner in that first round of fecal testing was our baby, Ami. Her microbiome was populated by more than 80 percent *Bifidobacterium* and more than 4 percent *Lactobacillus*. This was to be expected for a young baby who hadn't been weaned from breast milk yet. *Bifidobacterium* and *Lactobacillus* are often baby's first colonists, with bifidobacteria (especially *B. breve* and *B. longum*) making up 74 to 99 percent of the gut microbiome and lactobacilli (including *L. salivarius*, *L. casei*, *L. reuteri*, *L. rhamnosus*) representing 4 percent or more of the gut bacteria in a breast-fed baby.

Ami had recently navigated the birth canal, where microbes, especially *Lactobacillus*, entered her via her nose, mouth, and other membranes. Some of those microbes went down into her intestines, where they continued to grow and colonize the new territory. They grew exponentially, and by the end of her first week outside the womb there would have been more than 90 trillion. It was a land grab, but a welcome one. By populating and dominating the gut, millions of bifidobacteria and lactobacilli break down food into nutrients and fatty acids we can't make or process on their own, and they also edge out microbes that cause disease.

A few days after Ami's birth, the Bifs would have arrived in my breast milk. Awake to hormonal signals, they slip out of the maternal gut wall in the bloodstream, enter the lymph nodes, and from there flow to the mammary glands and into the milk. (Babies fed formula with a cow- or goat-milk base also have *Bifidobacterium*-dominated guts, although have about 20 percent less than babies fed human milk.)

Breast milk itself contains fifty-something sugars, called human milk oligosaccharides, that may exist solely to feed Bifs. Each woman makes her own bespoke sugar mix (determined by her genes, diet, and other factors), which is an important biological factoid to note, because certain species and subspecies of gut microbes flourish on certain sugars and not on others. A mom might hope that the sugars in her milk support species that are superior soothers. Ami, who's still breast-feeding at one year old, has always been a calm and alert baby. Maybe my milk sugar mix supports species of gut bugs that are especially effective at inducing calm. It's a lovely thought, and there may even be some truth to it.

But can her no-longer-breast-fed older sister catch up? Before I deliberately introduce Bifs and Lacts to my children, I wanted to know three things: what the microbes are doing, how they're doing it, and what motivates them.

Everything that's supposedly caused by stress, I tell people there's a Nobel Prize there if you find out the real cause. —Barry Marshall

The first thing that becomes clear in my investigation is that microbes are not martyrs. *Bifidobacterium* and *Lactobacillus* don't live to make us calmer and happier. It's the other way around: they make us calmer and happier so that they may live. These genera are especially sensitive to anxiety in their human hosts. When we're stressed, they die. The more anxious a mother is during pregnancy, the less *Lactobacillus* in her vagina, which means less *Lactobacillus* in the new baby. The more shaken a mom is during the postpartum months of nursing, the fewer Bifs in her breast milk. At exam time, when students are stressed out, their *Lactobacillus* count crashes, as several studies have shown. Tumult in the mind means tumult in the gut.

Over evolutionary time, the theory goes, *Bifidobacterium* and *Lactobacillus*, among other microbes, have developed tools to make us, their host and habitat, a more peaceful place so that they may have a better chance of surviving and thriving. How do they calm us? How do they hack us? Consider these sneaky strategies.

First, microbes tinker with our immune system as hackers might tinker with a burglar alarm. Over the eons, species of *Lactobacillus* and *Bifidobacterium* living in the gut wall have become especially adept at flipping genetic switches and dialing down activity in the immune cells they encounter. (Other species living in the respiratory system may do the same.) Sounds creepy, but you want this for your kid. Without this microbial tuning early in life, the immune system overreacts to anything it encounters just as an oversensitive security system does when the wind blows or the family cat enters the space. The term for this is inflammation, and the immune system in inflammatory mode is likelier to go after anything, friend or foe and in between. Inflammation in the gut wipes out microbes such as Bifs and Lacts, so they have a vested interest in helping us tamp it down.

A short word about inflammation, because it affects resilience and grit. Inflammation is what happens when white blood cells race to the site of a problem, like a sore throat or the lining of the lungs or intestines, to kill an infection and repair damaged tissue. Inflammatory molecules trigger pain fibers. It's a crucial immune response; without it, infections would fester and we wouldn't heal. But if inflammation is prolonged or too severe, healthy cells are damaged. Long-term low-level inflammation is linked with asthma, a higher risk of Type II diabetes, and many other diseases.

Inflammation may also be a mood killer. Proinflammatory cytokines, proteins produced by white blood cells, may indirectly prevent us from producing the neurotransmitter serotonin, which helps us feel calm. They also alter the production of dopamine, a hormone that helps keep us motivated. A chronic, systemic presence of these (testy, trigger-happy) soldiers might lead to a kid (or adult) feeling peevish, on edge, and less gratified for her efforts. If "good-guy" gut microbes were to prevent or reduce inflammation, the theory goes, the outcome would be a better baseline for mental health.

Bifidobacterium and *Lactobacillus* can also prevent inflammation from happening in the first place. When they (and other lactic-acid-producing gut bacteria) break down or ferment the food we eat, they leave behind a sort of gooey fatty-acid sludge. The sludge is full of nutrients that we can digest; the microbes have broken down the fiber for us. Just as important, the sludge coats the walls of our colon and intestines, sort of like the sealant that goes on leather. As a result, "bad" microbes don't leak into the bloodstream, where they might trigger chronic (mood-dampening, anxiety-inducing) inflammation throughout the body and even the brain.

The sludge is a gift that keeps on giving. Upon closer examination it also turns out to be rich in mind-modulating neurotransmitters: serotonin, dopamine, oxytocin, acetylcholine, and GABA (gamma-aminobutyric acid). These chemicals have sway over the behaviors that pretty much sum up who we are: what motivates us, what we find painful, and how much we bounce back. Generally speaking, serotonin and GABA soothe and relax, dopamine motivates, oxytocin bonds, and acetylcholine stimulates. So complex and potent is the alchemy in the gut that Justin Sonnenburg, a microbiology professor at Stanford, calls the compounds made by microbes an "unregulated pharmacy."

Looking at *Lactobacillus*, the discovery that it produces GABA is significant, because it's the GABA receptors in the brain that anti-anxiety drugs like Valium and Xanax target. (Some researchers think *Lactobacillus* is just as effective.) Specific species such as *L. reuteri* increase the number of cells in the brain that make oxytocin, the neurotransmitter released in touching, kissing, and bonding. *L. salivarius* and *L. farciminas*, meanwhile, have been found to decrease stress hormone (corticosteroid) production.

How might these signals from the gut reach the brain? Some microbes or their chemical compounds simply leave the gut and breach the blood-brain barrier. But in recent years, science has uncovered a more covert route: the vagus nerve, which extends its meandering way from the one hundred million digestive cells in the intestines to the brainstem by way of the heart, esophagus, and lungs, among other points of interest. Chemical signals produced by microbes go up the vagus, pass through the brain's switching station, and proceed from there to regions of the brain involved in neurotransmitter production or activity. Snip the vagus nerve, as scientists have done to lab mice, and those receptors don't receive, say, *Lactobacillus*'s calming signals from the gut below. (Signals also go down the vagus nerve from the brain to the gut, which is why distress causes stomach upset.)

Each genus, and even each species or subspecies, of microbe may have its own specialized brain-hacking toolkit. We know from Cryan's work, for instance, that *Lactobacillus* and *Bifidobacterium* seem to use different mechanisms to pull our strings. It's not much of a stretch to imagine that, for each of us, the balance of specific types in our guts, underlies our capacity for stress resilience. After all, their survival depends it.

A child's mind is not a container to be filled but rather a fire to be kindled. —Dorothea Brande

The next thing I wanted to know before putting my children on a *Bifidobacterium*- and *Lactobacillus*-heavy diet is what the buggers are supposed to do to the developing brain. Not just the young adult brain; I wanted to know about the infant or child's brain. The science here is very new, and so much is unknown, but there are a couple of tantalizing discoveries that open the frontier.

The first one that struck me stresses the role of *Lactobacillus* early in life or even before birth. Tracy Bale, a neuroscientist at the University of Pennsylvania, looked at the brains of normal mice versus mice that lacked *Lactobacillus*, and in the latter group she found unusual changes in the activity of more than twenty genes that affect brain development and function. Some of those altered genes code for new neurons and synapses in the hypothalamus, where the stress hormone cortisol is released. This finding suggests that *Lactobacillus* plays a role in modulating the HPA-axis, the body's response to stress. Extreme stress during pregnancy, Bale found, may alter the mother's vaginal microbiome, killing off lactobacilli that would normally transfer to her baby—and perhaps altering the activity of the baby's genes. (The latest trend is to swab the mother's vagina after a C-section birth and inoculate the baby orally, a method that achieves higher counts of healthy bacteria.) Indeed, some studies have found that newborns with low *Lactobacillus* counts are, on the whole, more distressed and colicky than their peers. (The jury is still out on whether it helps to feed them probiotic supplements.) Bale's work may help explain the heredity of stress: why children whose mothers were extremely frazzled during pregnancy also tend to be anxious.

Another mind-blowing discovery I came across concerns the role that *Lactobacillus* and *Bifidobacterium* (along with other fatty-acid fermenters) play in sculpting a child's brain. Yes, the physical struc-ture. In a nutshell, the psychobiotic fatty acids made by microbes target microglia, the brain's immune cells whose job it is to prune synapses, eat up dead neurons, and fight viruses, among other gar-dening and defense duties. When the gut microbiome is intact and diverse, microglia work as they should, regulating inflammation just enough to respond to pathogens. But when gut microbes have been wiped out or their diversity reduced, as they were in baby lab mice, the microglia in the brain become overactive and abnormal. The brain becomes inflamed, and if this goes on long enough, the microglia end up on a rampage, wiping out the synapses and neurons they're meant to protect.

Note that brain inflammation doesn't show up as the pain, swelling, or discomfort you'd experience when other body parts are inflamed. But it may contribute to fuzzy thinking, anxiety, depression, or behavioral downshifts like testiness, fussiness and—by extension—a loss of stress resilience. Happily, when gut microbiome diversity in mice was restored, their microglia became healthy again. (See chapter 2 for ways to increase gut microbiome diversity.)

Microglia, it turns out, are especially important during developmental windows in the early years and in adolescence, when they prune back synapses, rewire connections, and essentially remodel the brain for the next life stage. You want that pruning process to go well: don't cut too much or too little; remove the dead connections and reorganize the important ones. The outcome depends on the health of microglia—which, by extension, may depend a lot on the health of the gut microbes. What hangs in the balance is how vulnerable a child will be to anxiety, depression, and other psychiatric conditions later in life. We need science to look especially closely at the impact of antibiotics on the infant and teenage brain.

So with all this, the mystery of microbial mind control deepens even as it is better understood. The takeaway is that microbes can hack our brains in several ways: by dialing down anxiety-inducing inflammation caused by an oversensitive immune system; by preventing infection, thereby subverting inflammation; by sending signals to the brain up the vagus nerve or through the blood-brain barrier, altering hormone and neurotransmitter levels; and by shaping the brain structures involved in cognition and the stress response. Some microbe hacks may hurt us, but many clearly help us.

My family will settle for any and all routes to resilience.

Tell me and I forget; Teach me and I remember; Involve me and I learn. —Benjamin Franklin (attributed)

Now the next burning question: How much, in a month or so, can you increase your child's population of bifidobacteria and lactobacilli—and, if you raise it significantly, what will happen? I prep UJ for the undertaking by talking up "Bifs" and "Lacts." "They're soothers,"

I say. I whip out my smartphone and show her what they look like under a microscope. *Bifidobacterium* look like twigs (from the Latin *bifidus*, "to fork") and *Lactobacillus* (from *lacto*, "milk," and *baci*, "rod") look like puffy pills, but they're both basically tubular bits and pieces. I call them peaceniks. "Cute!" she chirps. The two go together in a sort of singsong: *Bifs and Lacts and Lacts and Bifs and Lacts and Bifs and Bifs and Lacts . . .*

"Here's the deal," I say as I stir a pot of warm milk for home-made yogurt. "You get to eat a bowlful of this twice a day, morning and snack." Technically, I want my daughters to eat two eight-ounce servings of yogurt a day (along with other microbe-filled foods) for at least four weeks. That's the regimen in most of the studies that we're using to model our informal experiment. The scientists behind these studies are often conservative, saying that there's still too much that we don't know about how and why they work, and for whom. But the risk is low (these are microbes that humans have hosted for millennia) and the potential upside is high, so why not? UJ gives a sort of comic groan, then nods.

We eat homemade yogurt and supplement it with brands like Stonyfield and Maple Hills Farms, plain, with no added sugars, gela-tin, or other fillers. The homemade yogurt begins with a freeze-dried mail-order starter culture. On the premise that some peaceniks may be more effective than others, I chose starters with the species used in studies: *B. breve*, *B. longum*, and *B. animalis* (spp. *Lactis*), and *L. bulgaricus*, *L. casei*, and *L. helveticus*. Most cultures contain multiple species. UJ's fecal samples from her test the previous year were low to nil in these species. Will they show up on the next test?

In a cold winter kitchen, a yogurt maker is a warm spot. My husband, Peter, becomes the self-appointed yogurt chef, a throwback to his college days at Berkeley. To my surprise, Ami loves the sour-ish stuff, and baby signs for more. Picky UJ eats it, too. We doctor it with blueberry jam or honey, walnuts, and muesli. Sometimes, we stir in a spoonful of the supersweet mango lassi from the Indian restaurant around the corner. Yogurt becomes a smoothie-booster. It's a breakfast, a side dish, an after-school snack. Once, to the frank disappointment of all, it is dessert.

Most of the Bifs and Lacts will just pass through the intestines and colon without sticking around, I tell UJ with a shrug. But if she eats enough often enough, they may have a calming influence on her as they go by, like a choir walking down a city street. If she eats oats and garlic, onions and other supportive fibers that Bifs and Lacts feed on, the "choir" may stick around longer. Kefir, for instance, includes healthy yeasts, which are known to give *Lactobacillus* better staying power. Dark chocolate and foods containing oligosaccharides also help increase bifidobacteria and lactobacilli in the gut (see more tips in text box). Whether and for how long the microbes will hang out in her gut, or anyone's, depends on genes, timing, stress, the other gut microbes present, and especially whatever else she eats to support them.

The good news from oddball randomized trials keeps our yogurt maker warm. One study recruited die-hard smokers and found that kefir, chock-full of *Lactobacillus*, gave them the grit to finally quit. In another, farm-raised tilapia, which usually go belly-up due to stress from overcrowding, survived and seemingly thrived with a *Lactobacillus* supplement in their feed. Another study set out to prove that the microbes have mind-control properties and fed nervous mice the microbes from easygoing resilient mice. Guess what happened? The nervous mice became resilient too. A gut microbe transplant was nothing short of a personality transplant. Astonishing.

Then, most optimistic of all, this one. In a small trial at UCLA led by Kirsten Tillisch, women ate a probiotic yogurt like ours twice daily. One month later, fMRI scans revealed that areas of their brains related to stress were altered. Compared to a control group, the yogurt eaters' insula—an area of the brain that processes sensations from the gut and other areas—showed greater connectivity in areas of the prefrontal cortex involved in decision-making and control. When the subjects in the study were shown threatening images, the control group immediately felt anxious while the yogurt eaters' brains stayed chill and relaxed—because they weren't anticipating something stressful or alarming. One explanation that Tillisch and her colleagues offer is that the microbes in the yogurt reduced inflammatory cytokines, and less inflammation leads to improved brain activity and mood.

There are real-world applications here for our kids. Imagine a difficult test is coming down the pike. For medical students who participated in a gut microbe study in Japan, it was the nationwide exam. Beginning eight weeks before the test, student volunteers drank a daily serving of either a placebo or a fermented milk cultured with a strain of *Lactobacillus casei*. The day before the exam the students that unknowingly took the placebo reported feeling much more anxious and had higher cortisol levels than the *L. casei* group.

All this suggests a real boost in stress resilience for those who take *Lactobacillus*. In the last four weeks before the test, the microbe-boosted students also had only one-third as many stomachaches, colds, or runny noses as the untreated students. Bonus.

Biohack: Homemade Grit

Take on this experiment with a growth mindset. The idea is that a healthy gut community with a lot of lactic-acid-making gut bacteria may help children bounce back better and decrease their baseline anxiety. It must be said that there's no known ideal amount of *Lactobacillus* or *Bifidobacterium* in the body, much less an ideal-for-all-guts species or strain; there are too many unknowns. But we're not taking a lot of risks by eating two 8-ounce servings of yogurt daily. These probiotic foods have been part of the human diet for thousands of years.

While a yogurt maker isn't compulsory, it's convenient because it keeps the yogurt warmed to the right temperature for the hours it needs to culture. (A slow cooker works too.) Here's what we did:

1. Buy yogurt starter capsules that include the species (if not the exact subspecies) used in scientific experiments: *Lactobacillus* (including *L. rhamnosus*, *L. reuteri*, and *L. helveticus*) and *Bifidobacterium* (including *B. breve* and *B. longum*). Note: You can't predict if all the species are going to thrive equally well in a homemade culture, or if a handful will dominate. We get what we get (with the goal of not getting upset).

2. Heat up 1 liter of milk (cow milk or soy; not ultrapasteurized) or whole milk yogurt to 180°F for two minutes to kill off bacteria that could compete with your culture, then let it cool to 115°F before whisking in one to two capsules.

3. Pour the mixture into a sealable container (yogurt maker). Incubate the mix at around 100°F for six to ten hours. Optional: put aside ½ cup in a glass jar in the fridge to use as a starter next time (1 tablespoon per liter).

4. Add grit to your diet separately. If you put goldfish in a tank and you want them to live, you'll need to give them fish food, and the same goes for microbes. Put Bifs and Lacts in the kid's tank, and then feed them simple sugars that might not be in the regular diet. By this I mean 5 grams of the microbes' favorite prebiotic fibers: fructooligosaccharide (FOS) and galactooligosaccharide (GOS). In one study, a GOS supplement given to children at a dose of 2 grams per day doubled the population of *Bifidobacterium* over three weeks compared to a placebo. The result: kids who took the GOS had significantly reduced cortisol in the morning, suggesting a lower stress response, and an increased focus on cheery images in an

emotional processing task. (Caveat: this was industry-funded research.) For natural prebiotics, eat more fiber.

FOS and GOS are available in capsule form online and can be cooked or frozen in food without compromising their health properties. Arguably, it's better to get your GOS and FOS naturally in onions, garlic, milk, bananas, wheat, oats, artichokes, and asparagus. Of note, dark chocolate, and the polyphenols in it, supports growth of both *Bifidobacterium* and *Lactobacillus*.

Homemade yogurt can also be made from alternative nondairy milks, including cashew, coconut, hemp, rice, sunflower seed, soy, and almond. These milks may require the addition of a thickener such as pectin when the culture is added.

Be wary of *probiotic* pills. When microbes are consumed in pill form, even in the freeze-dried billions, they're less likely to survive stomach acids or stick around in the intestines. When probiotics are eaten in food, however, the good microbes are likelier to survive their trip to the intestinal tract and set up residence. (Research finds this is especially true when delivered in a dairy product.) Fermented foods such as kimchi, pickles, and miso are also high in *Lactobacillus*. (We add miso to soup and pastas, which also adds a touch of umami je ne sais quoi.) Eat prebiotics and probiotics together for serious symbiotic perks.

I should add a commonsensical caveat here. Every person's internal ecosystem is different. Bifs and Lacts have lived in us for eons, but if your child doesn't respond well to probiotic foods (gets diarrhea or becomes constipated, bloated, or feverish), stop the diet. For instance, it's known that some strains of *Lactobacillus* can exacerbate the symptoms of chronic fatigue syndrome sufferers, perhaps by overstimulating the immune response and causing inflammation.

For gut microbiota sequencing, there are two popular services: American Gut, a crowd-sourced citizen scientist project (www .americangut.org), and uBiome, a California biotech company (www.ubiome.com). A newer service, Viome (www.viome.com), offers a more thorough form of microbiome sequencing that identifies bacteria as well as other gut microbes, including viruses, parasites, yeast, and fungi, and identifies chemical byproducts of gut microorganisms.

Bifs and Lacts and Lacts and Bifs. How are we doing? One blustery sleet-gray day at the end of the month I sent out the children's fecal samples to the lab for a "post-intervention" test. After weeks of intensive yogurt consumption with prebiotics, I am hopeful that I'll see UJ's counts rise from where they had been in the test last spring. On the behavioral front, however, I can report no transfiguring cataclysmic change. We are not experiencing a light-stricken moment of life-changing awe. There is no light streaming down from the heavens, nor a golden path to bliss rolling out before us. The Earth is still round. And bitter cold.

But there are glimmers of something around the third week of the experiment, the same time frame when a shift started to happen in Cryan's and Tillisch's studies. UJ's school holds an ice skating party in the park. This is her first time on skates, and she is terribly unsteady. Several kids her age, five or six, take to the ice right away. In a heartbreaking moment, I witness my daughter's expression as two girls in her class link arms and take off, giggling, just like that. Every time UJ slips and falls, she drags herself up to her knees, then her feet, one massive skate at a time. The klieg lights intensify the moment, like the lights of a high-powered microscope, and I feel as if we were struggling in an icy petri dish. After a while, UJ pushes away my helping hand. *Stop. Get away, I can do it myself.* I stand on the ice alone, watching with pain and pride as my daughter falls, gets up, falls, gets up again, alone, until the kliegs click off.

Back home, little Ami, now almost exactly one year old, also shoves my hand away. She's learning to walk. She falls, gets up, falls, and falls again. "By self! Self! Self only!" Down and up and down and up.

The same could be said for the lab results when they eventually arrive. One's down, one's up. After a month of special yogurt, Ami's population of *Bifidobacterium* and *Lactobacillus* have fallen hard, down to about 5 percent of her sample. I remind myself that counts can shift daily. Sometimes a discrepancy like this arises because results vary between labs and there's no standardization. But the likely reason is that the child now eats solids whereas before, during the earlier test, she was on a breast milk only diet. Even babies that were stuffed with Bifs and Lacts, as Ami was nine months ago, won't necessarily have much of those microbes left after those first mouthfuls of peas and bananas. The gut microbiota diversifies and becomes more complex until sometime between ages three and five. So, for her, the relatively smaller population of these two microbes is a sign that her diversity has boomed. Around UJ's age, six, the population stabilizes more, although the proportion of one species relative to others may seesaw dramatically even within a day (especially after antibiotics, sickness, stress, travel, or a dietary intervention).

UJ gets a high-five for her results. Thanks to the yogurt experiment, *Bifidobacterium* represents up to 6 percent of her sample, and *Lactobacillus* around 2 percent. UJ's Bifs, the report suggests, are more than twice as high as that of the average American. When I drill down to the species level, I see *B. longum* and *B. breve* are present; these are the highly desirable types associated with calm and longevity that were used in studies and are in the homemade yogurt. Not a trace of them had been detected in the earlier tests. We're going in the right direction (although, of course, percentages can vary with every meal). UJ takes in this news quietly. Her good guys aren't exactly overcoming, but they're rising up.

Whatever this means, who can tell for sure? There are signs of grit in both children, maybe more than before, but it's hard to know what to credit: development, focused parenting, better communication, the season? Maybe, for UJ, it was the microbes—or just the expectation that the Bifs and Lacts might help her persevere. Neither child fell ill those weeks—all the yogurt and kefir in their diet may have boosted immunity, and health itself is stress resilience, right? Perhaps the real value of the experiment is that we're all paying more attention. In the end, what matters is that when the kids fall, they rise up again.

And so it comes to pass that, three weeks after Martin Luther King Jr. Day and five weeks into our experiment, UJ is practicing her violin as usual. Outside, the trees are bare and handfuls of icy snow spatter on the windows. She plays the same wrong note twice. She skips a whole section of a song, something she hadn't done for a while. I act on an inexplicable urge to straighten her wrist. My correction triggers an outburst, and soon enough, child and violin are on the floor.

"Are we done?" I ask in a fed-up monotone. This parent might need more yogurt.

She looks up at me with a fierce new expression. "Mama. When I'm stopping, I don't mean I'm quitting." She stands up and tucks the violin in her armpit. "I mean *pausing*. Only for a little while, Mama, not forever. Like a *fermata*, Mama." Then, with a blotchy face and trembling bow hold, she resumes her playing.

Fermata. It sounds like ferment. I look up what it means in musical notation: *sustain this longer than its normal duration would indicate.*

FEBRUARY

On Gut Bugs and
Social Butterflies

Can diet affect social life?

A CHILD CANNOT THRIVE on yogurt alone, but that's about the healthiest food my elder daughter now eats regularly. Of the many humbling blunders I've made as a mother, perhaps the biggest is UJ's diet. My firstborn started out strong enough on breast milk—eighteen months of it! But like most American kids, the color of her diet never sufficiently progressed from whites and beiges to the full rainbow. The kid overwhelmingly prefers pasta, crackers, tofu, and white-flour tortillas. If nudged she'll eat eggs, walnuts, and salmon, but somehow two pescetarian (fish eating but otherwise vegetarian) parents have managed to raise a child that finds fruit and veggies more appalling than appealing.

When Ami came along four and a half years later, I vowed to give her a rainbow diet from the start. Because this baby was introduced to solid food in the summer, her first fruits and vegetables weren't the winter-pale ones that UJ ate at that age, but the cream of the high-summer farmer's market. I've wondered if this more favorable initial exposure made a difference later. Whereas UJ had spit out her first winter squash purees, her carrot mash, and her spinach-turnip soups, Ami devoured her watermelon, her raspberries, her graffiti eggplant rollatini. Her first tomatoes were of the vine-ripened heirloom variety; her first strawberries and blueberries were wild and handpicked by me; and then came garden peas, sweet summer corn, backyard broccoli. Later came yogurt and high-fiber hot cereal with banana and blackberries; sardines and egg with unpeeled pear. Even now, in the winter, she eats almost everything.

Ami's grinning mouth always has a sticky ring of fruit juice and flaxseed or dried blueberry around it. "She looks so self-satisfied," a family friend observed.

She is. Ami is also a risk-taker, a charmer, an independent spirit with a question mark of downy hair sticking up. Make a sudden loud noise and she'll startle—then smile and sign (finger to palm) for more. In the bathtub, she likes to slip neatly under the water, belly-up and fish-eyed, until I swoop in, horrified, for this is exactly how she'd look if she'd drowned. She breathes in, gasping, and breathes out, laughing, amusement in her impish brown eyes. She makes smiley eye contact with strangers on the subway. Hold her and she molds to your body.

Our firstborn was just as sweet when she was a baby, if not sweeter, and remains so much of the time. But she was more sensitive and sometimes suspicious of novelty. In preschool, UJ would often spend free time alone, in a crate on the blacktop, watching the other toddlers. She prefers individuals to groups. She's subtle. She doesn't want to be a follower, she says, of the classroom bully who is making everyone a servant at recess time. On Valentine's Day this month, she writes a nuanced card to the girl. "I appreciate you for saying you're sorry when you're mean." And seals it with a heart.

"While genes are pivotal in establishing some aspects of emotionality," wrote the doctor and researcher Thomas Lewis, "experience plays a central role in turning genes on and off. The genetic lottery may determine the cards in your deck, but experience deals the hand you can play." It sounds implausible, but science has begun to ask the controversial question about whether the gut microbiome qualifies as a life experience that tweaks a person's temperament and emotional responses. Is it possible that the most sociable, well-adjusted kids have different microbiomes from the shyest kids? Is there a microbial signature for an extroverted, risk-taking personality? If so, is it coincidence or could the bugs tinker with temperament? So much food for thought.

I'm very shy so I became very outgoing to protect my shyness.
—Don Rickles

Given the gastronomic and temperamental differences between my two girls, I wasn't surprised when news broke that microbiologists from the Ohio State University Institute for Behavioral Medicine Research found correlations between social behavior and gut microbiota. In a nutshell, the principal researchers, Lisa Christian and Michael Bailey, had asked about eighty moms of two-year-olds to assess their child's temperament: How excited does the child get when presented with a new toy? How fussy does the kid get with a new babysitter? How quickly does the toddler recover from a bump or scrape? How negatively does the child respond when she doesn't get her way? When playing outdoors, how often does he make a lot of noise or stray from Mama or want to climb to high places? Bailey and Christian then tested each child's diaper-salvaged stool sample for the type and number of microbes within.

Tick the boxes yourself. Is your child basically self-assured? Upbeat? Sociable? Dominant? Talkative? Assertive? Enthusiastic? Sensation-seeking? Impulsive? Engaged in his or her environment? What Christian and Bailey found was that kids who had these traits associated with extraversion/surgency were likelier than others to have a greater diversity of bacterial species in their gut. In other words, the most outgoing and buoyant kids had the most cosmopolitan microbiome with a greater-than-average presence of unique species. The fewer species of microbes in a child's stool sample, the less outgoing, risk-taking, and curious the kid (generally, of course). Coincidence or not?

Between my two children, you might guess that the toddler with the complex, high-fiber, veggie-heavy diet would have the greater diversity of microbes in her gut, and you'd be right. My finicky eldest with the pasta predilection had lower-than-average gut microbiota diversity in her first test (although her diversity had increased after last month's yogurt eating). It's possible that her pickiness was perpetuated by a bacterial imbalance, with certain dominant species sending starchy high-carb-jonesing signals to the brain, in the absence of veggie- and high-fiber-loving bacteria to offset them.

UJ's gut microbiome diversity wasn't dreadfully low, but imagine the following: A forest has ten thousand trees in it. If all ten thousand trees are pines, there's no diversity, just pines. That's not UJ—she has more variety than that. But if her gut were a forest in autumn, it's fair to say that it wouldn't make for the most spectacular fall foliage tour. Compare that to a forest in which there's a lot of variety among the ten thousand trees—the usual pines along with maples and oaks, as well as redwoods, ash, bamboo, and, say, some exotic species such as baobab and silk cotton. This is extreme diversity, and although neither of my children's results qualified as extreme in either direction, my younger daughter's gut microbiome was generally more diverse than her sister's. Ami has the usual array of common microbes: a lot of *Bacteroides* and some Firmicutes, *Prevotella* and Proteobacteria. But she also hosts some rare species found in no other member of the family. (Note: An infant's gut microbiome is often surprisingly low in diversity because bifidobacteria dominate in breast milk–fed babies, a profile linked with the best health and cognitive outcomes. Diversity generally increases as new foods are introduced and the milk-fed microbiome is shouldered out, but Ami's results would bounce around a lot between her first and second birthdays.)

Going by Christian and Bailey's study, it fits that Ami is more of an assertive, energetic babbler than her sister. The experiment's high-diversity group tended to be more "Extraverted and Surgent" than the low-diversity group. They were more likely to be described as active, bold, dominant, joyful, and energetic. In boys, a high diversity of gut microbes was particularly associated with two subcategories of personality traits: sociability (personal warmth) and high-intensity pleasure. If there's a rope web to climb, the high-surgency kid will clamber to the mosh pit center, even if older kids are manically jumping around there. At preschool, the extroverted/surgent kid is likelier to quickly befriend other kids. If there's a fountain to run through, the surgent kid may run over and drench herself without much pause for reflection. Yes, that's more like my secondborn.

Kids whose gut microbiota were low in biodiversity also shared a few striking similarities. The girls enjoyed cuddling with their parents more than did kids with more diversity. These low-diversity daughters also had more self-restraint, which describes my firstborn (and I wouldn't necessarily want to change that). In other research, kids with low gut microbiota diversity were less physically fit and heavier. Remember, this was a more cautious group, so perhaps they seek physical comfort more, are less active, and are better able to resist temptation. Bailey's team found no other noteworthy differences between boys and girls in the types and abundance of microbiota. What they did find, however, was that the correlation between microbiota and temperament persisted even when they took into consideration how the child was delivered—vaginally or surgically—and whether or not he or she was breast-fed.

So, there it is. Young children who seem generally more optimistic and extroverted have lots of diverse gut microbes, while those who seem less surgent and sociable have less diversity (at least in this body of research). Sounds straightforward enough, but if you think about it, there are a few chicken-and-egg problems to ponder. Does gut biodiversity *drive* a kid to act bolder or more sociably? Or is a diverse gut microbiome just a biomarker of a happy, healthy, outgoing kid with good genes and more openness to healthy food? Maybe kids on the sociable side of the spectrum are more easygoing in some ways, including in their willingness to eat healthy pre- and probiotic foods. In other words, do the microbes influence the behavior, or does the behavior influence the microbes?

What comes first, the social butterfly or the egg?

Are we in charge, or are we simply hosts for bacteria?
It all depends on your outlook. —Neil deGrasse Tyson

Remember John Cryan? He's the neuroscientist who found that *Lactobacillus* and *Bifidobacterium* correlate with a decrease in anxiety and an increase in resilience. Cryan has built a case for the little guys. If you're a microbe, he claims, you have an ulterior motive for making your human host get along with others. The more extroverted your chump is, the more contact he or she has with others, and the more likely it is that your kind will get a chance to spread to new hosts. You might help your host increase hormones that attract her to others, or others to her, which would ensure that microbes like you will have more hosts to live in. For instance, certain species such as *L.reuteri* may stimulate the production of oxytocin, a hormone associated with cooperation and social gratification.

As fantastical and farfetched as that sounds, the idea is that the most sociable people (and other hosts) may harbor a greater kind or variety of microbes that enhance sociability and intimacy, which in turn treat the microbes to increased contact with new bodies to occupy. After all, each of us releases our own personal microbial cloud, shedding 10^6 particles an hour, including *Lactobacillus*, which may, over time, colonize other people. (Yes, long-term contact can help shape the gut microbiome.) In adults, certain microbes or microbial mixes may increase the possibility of attracting a mate, which could lead to a new host in the form of a baby. Cryan floats the idea that microbes in the intestinal walls may act on our cells to produce molecules that act on neural signaling, which would tune sociability, mood, and other aspects of behavior.

Consider, too, the evidence that suggests that microbes help to wire the social brain in its earliest stages. It begins with the observation that microbe-free mice raised in germ-free conditions all their lives are basically unadventurous and unsociable. If they see another mouse in another chamber, they avoid it—and that's weird for a mouse. There's no sense of a stable social community among microbe-free mice. Their social impairments remind researchers of autism.

Perhaps not coincidentally kids with autism tend to have less diverse gut microbiomes than the norm (as well as fewer fermenters like *Lactobacillus* that help seal the gut), although the cause is unclear. Children whose mothers took antibiotics in pregnancy are likelier to have autism. These moms would have had less gut biodiversity while pregnant, and the absence of certain microbes might have had an impact on the fetal brain. One study found that it takes four months for the average person to regain gut microbiome diversity after taking the common antibiotic clindamycin. It takes up to a year after a round of the broad-spectrum bomb Cipro. (Is it possible that kids who had taken frequent rounds of antibiotics, especially the kinds that cause long-term loss of gut biodiversity, are less sociable? Would a diet with probiotics and high-fiber foods have offset any impact? That study has yet to be done.)

The dream is that microbiome research on unsociable mice might lead to therapies for human social disorders. Some of these studies have made people immensely hopeful. In one, researchers cultured *Lactobacillus reuteri* from human breast milk and transferred it to socially deficient bacteria-free mice after weaning. As if by divine intervention, those mice started acting as friendly and curious as normal mice. How? *L. reuteri* is known to trigger the production of oxytocin, a bonding hormone that improves sociability and mood by sending antianxiety signals up the vagus nerve. In another mouse study, a species of *Bifidobacterium*, *B. fragiles*, was introduced, again reversing unsociable behavior, so it seems that more than one kind of microbe can influence a rodent's social warmth and curiosity—and likely ours, too. (Autism is a much more complex condition in humans than in mice. Altering the gut microbiome may help alleviate some undesirable autism-related behavior, but only for a certain percent of the population.)

In autism research *B. fragiles* and *L. reuteri* get a lot attention, but they aren't the only stars of the show. Microbes produce untold combinations of neurotransmitters and neuromodulators that could influence their host's social warmth and motivation. Gut bacteria themselves are social and symbiotic critters; they live off one another's by-products; they have friends and foes; they communicate with one another and form pacts. The gut is a community, a culture.

Looking at the pantheon of microbes in our guts, which ones so far have proven themselves to be the best tinkerers? Here's a quick roll call:

- Species of *Lactobacillus* and *Bifidobacterium* produce GABA, which has a calming, stabilizing effect on the brain that could reduce social anxiety. *Lactobacillus* also produces acetylcholine, which boosts spirits and synaptic flexibility and keeps bad moods and aggression in check. By itself, acetylcholine has been found to help social deficiency (and reduce cognitive inflexibility, another autism trait) in lab mice. A large study of more than seven hundred young adults found that consumption of fermented food containing *Lactobacillus* and other beneficial microbes—a diet that includes kefir, sauerkraut, pickles, kimchi, and the like—was specifically linked to significantly reduced social anxiety. That is, people who normally scored highest in neuroticism—for instance, feeling shy at a gathering or around unfamiliar faces, or fearful of being judged or called on in class, or worried that they'll embarrass themselves—were somewhat protected by having *Lactobacillus* and other microbes in their diet.

- *Bacillus*, *Saccharomyces*, and *Escherichia* produce norepinephrine, which triggers the fight-or-flight response but also enhances the experience of joy, depending on degree and context. When norepinephrine levels are low, we feel sluggish and depressed, with little interest in other people.

- Then there's *Streptococcus*, *Escherichia*, and *Enterococcus* spp., along with species of *Lactobacillus*, *Bifidobacterium*, and *Lactococcus*, which are all involved in the production of soothing serotonin or serotonin receptors (5-HT) in the brain and throughout the nervous system, including the vagus nerve. Serotonin influences everything from anxiety to aggression, memory to mood. (More isn't always better: an excess of gut-sourced serotonin may be detrimental, and some species, like *E. coli* and *S. pharyngitus*, are pathogens).

How do these guys get to our controls? Again, some send signals up the vagus nerve from the gut, triggering the production of neurotransmitters in the brain. When microbe-made neurotransmitters are in the bloodstream they can signal across the brain-blood barrier to the hypothalamus, which curbs the stress response (HPA axis). They can also tweak our behavior indirectly by reducing inflammation.

An idea that excites scientists working in child development is that different combinations of microbes early in life lead to different quantities of neurotransmitters like GABA and serotonin, which in turn sculpt the child's synapses and shape her temperament. Think about it. The cognitive resources that counter social threats (novelty, rejection, fear) or enhance social motivation require a whole arsenal of neurotransmitters and nervous system stabilizers.

If there's an argument for why gut microbiome diversity might be more important to mental health, it's this. The wider your variety of gut bugs, the larger your toolkit. You can see why kids with the most diverse biota-friendly diets may be better equipped to cope with whatever twists and turns they encounter in their social landscape.

Evil is a word we use to describe the absence of good.
—William Paul Young

Maybe it's not only the bugs we *have* that dial up a child's sociability—maybe it's also the *absence* of the ones that dial down sociability. Maybe "sociability" here is just a proxy for being well-adjusted and curious about and receptive to others. Germs, viruses, and toxins can make us less agreeable or less motivated, and diversity keeps those bad guys in check.

As the Environmental Protection Agency puts it, "The solution to pollution is dilution." Our own genes can't adapt and respond as quickly to change—intruders or adverse environmental conditions—but our gut microbes can. These little guys can replicate every six minutes or so, and they can mutate when necessary, which means they're very nimble and responsive under adversity. If you don't want kudzu to take over your garden, you're going to want a variety of adaptable, fast-growing acacia, pines, palms, lemongrass, and so on to crowd it out.

To demonstrate the power of an unchecked species, researchers at Texas Tech University transferred the "bad guy" microbe *Campylobacter jejuni* from anxious mice to a group of microbe-free mice. Without other gut microbes to make gut-sealing goo or kill the pathogen, *Campylobacter* can eat through the mucus layer in the gut wall and rupture it, which allows the bacteria or their neurotoxic by-products an easy escape into the bloodstream. Just two days later—an indication of how quickly the gut microbiome can change—the transplant recipients became diffident and socially avoidant. The resulting inflammation, if chronic, triggers a cascade of immune responses, including anxiety and unease. The stress also reduces biodiversity in the gut, allowing *C. jejuni* and other pathogens to dominate more than they would otherwise. It's a vicious cycle.

An overabundance of *Ruminococcus*, a microbe associated with a high-fat, high-sugar, low-fiber diet, may also harm the developing brain. This microbe may communicate with the brain via the hormone cortisol, found a group at the University of Illinois at Urbana-Champaign. Cortisol, in turn, controls a crucial brain chemical called n-acetylaspartate (NAA). Babies need NAA; it's a marker of mental health, creativity, reasoning, and fluid intelligence, and low levels are correlated with lower scores of intellectual function, anxiety disorders, and antisocial or autistic behavior. When baby pigs had an abundance of *Ruminococcus*, their cortisol levels were lower, leading to lower-than-average amounts of NAA in their brain. Much remains unknown about the *Ruminococcus* connection in humans, or why some infants have *Ruminococus*-dominant guts, but the suggestion that a gut microbiome imbalance may indirectly harm a baby's brain is as promising as it is disturbing.

In Bailey and Christian's study, girls who had the highest amount of *Rikenellaceae* (a family of microbes previously linked with depression) tended to be more fearful than average. Their moms rated them as uneasy and easily startled. *Rikenellaceae*, in excess, is also associated with a high-fat diet. One explanation is that when certain microbes such as this are out of whack, they may secrete neurotoxins when they break down manufactured foods, resulting in inflammation, and their distress signals go up the vagus nerve, causing low-grade anxiety. If there were a diversity of other microbes present, some would seal the gut and others would work together to kill, crowd out, or contain those renegade microbes.

Comparing the gut microbe test results of my two girls from the first to the second tests, I saw that my elder daughter's *Rikenellaceae* went from slightly above normal to normal for people of all ages. My fearless young daughter had lower than average levels of that species. I was also delighted to see that both girls had lower than average levels of inflammatory microbes such as *Enterobacter*, and the diversity of microbes in UJ's gut microbiome apparently increased from its modest baseline of a year ago.

As children's gut biodiversity increases, their social brains may be better protected from neurotoxins that have an impact on development—even at low levels. Everyday neurotoxins include the pesticides in our produce and parks; the BPA (bisphenol) in food packaging and paper products; the phthalates and parabens in fragrances, air fresheners, and cleaning agents; food dyes; fire retardants (PBDEs) in furniture, rug pads, and electronics; vehicle exhaust and fine particulate matter—they're are all linked with cognitive and social deficits, ADHD, and autism-spectrum disorders.

This winter, ornamental purple cabbage is growing at the apartment complex at our corner, and the groundskeepers doused it with nauseating quantities of high-phthalate air freshener to repel rats. We all breathe in the brain-numbing chemical as we pass the cabbages; small children also love to touch the ruffled leaves. Cabbage heads don't make children brain-dead, but over time, multiple exposures to multiple neurotoxins may lead to an ambient depression and low-level social problems that wouldn't show up clinically. They might just subtly nudge a kid toward being a bit more negative and less genial. Nothing that can be pinpointed, just a tiny shift. The more species of gut microbes that kids have, however, the better their Swiss army knife of defenses against the neurotoxins they encounter every day of their young lives.

After all, you never know which microbe, or which probiotic combo, might hit the jackpot or cure what ails. In a recent study, children fed probiotic yogurt containing our old friend *Lactobacillus rhamnosus* absorbed significantly less toxic heavy metals like mercury, arsenic, and lead into their bloodstream—all of which, even at a chronic low level, can lead to cognitive problems and social disorders. The bacteria block absorption or bind the metals, deactivate them, and flush them out of the system.

B. breve and *L. casei*, along with another microbe, *Bacillus pumilus*, found in kimchi, can degrade the endocrine disruptor BPA. Another gut microbe, *Burkholderia cepacia*, earned its keep in the broad-headed stinkbug by breaking down and eliminating pesticides so well that the insect could survive even after being bombed with some of the strongest chemicals available. (The microbe can also break down and remove contaminants from soil.)

Maybe the best way to think of the impact of the gut bug pantheon on our kids' social lives is in its ability to nudge. The microbiome is not a puppeteer; it's a nudge. It may nudge children to a better state of calm. It may nudge them toward stronger neurotoxin resistance and the ability to recover from everyday toxic exposures. It may nudge them toward stronger nervous system reflexes and an upbeat mood. It may nudge them toward better bounce back from adversity. All these tiny nudges have knock-on effects on energy, agreeableness, and positivity in how kids interact with other people. The best news, according to Cryan, is that microbes may continue to influence the developing nervous system well into adolescence. *It's not too late.*

The diversity of the phenomena of nature is so great, and the treasures hidden in the heavens so rich, precisely in order that the human mind shall never be lacking in fresh nourishment.
—Johannes Kepler

"The goal is to grow as many different types of good-guy bacteria inside you as possible," I tell UJ. "There's an easy way and there's a hard way to do it. What's your pick?"

"The easy way," she says with confidence.

"Great," I say. "Here's the plan. In Africa, there are hunter-gatherer people called the Hadza, and they eat a diet with a lot of fiber. Good-guy microbes love fiber, so you'll find a large variety of healthy microbes in their guts and in their poop. We'll ask a Hadza person for her poop, and we'll squirt it with all the good-guy microbes into your colon."

"My what?"

"Guess."

UJ looks at me in horror. It's true that the Hadza, a modern hunter-gatherer group living in Tanzania, have twice the gut microbiota diversity of the average American, thanks in part to their fiber-rich diet of tubers, seeds, and baobob and consumption of, say, raw zebra and monkey organs. They also have fewer inflammatory factors from gut metabolites than do people on a Western diet. (However, it's interesting to note that they have much less bifidobacteria post-weaning than we do; researchers suggest that this genus became adaptive after the introduction of agriculture and farming.) In theory, a fecal microbiota transplant of exotic Hadza bacteria would colonize a Western intestine, at least temporarily. (Anthropologist Jeff Leach, founder of American Gut and the Human Food Project, undertook this very experiment. An unsupervised fecal transplant is not actually recommended for many, many, many reasons, including the possibility of disease transmission.)

UJ blinks. "What! I will not!"

"OK, then you'll have to do your own chewing," I tell her.

It's true that if UJ eats a more diverse diet, she'll likely develop a more diverse microbiome. Diet accounts for up to 60 percent of the composition and characteristics of microbes in our intestines, and the population of any given species can go up and down in a flash depending on what we eat. Genes, meanwhile, are thought to influence no more than 12 percent of the gut microbiome, and the remaining 28 percent is attributed to environment, such as the soil and air, the people who live with us, sleep and exercise, and microbes acquired in early life.

Whether the fiber eater's sociability will increase along with her gut microbiota diversity is unknown. While it's possible that diet drives the associations that Bailey and Christian saw between the gut microbiome and personality, they could not prove it. The researchers asked mothers to remember the foods the subjects ate, but the survey didn't consider foods consumed over the long term, even though impressions of temperament are often formed early on. Nor did the study track fiber consumption, which boosts gut microbiome diversity. As always, more research is needed. How wonderful it would be, I thought, to have a randomized double-blind experiment in which subjects deliberately diversify their gut microbiota and researchers rate their sociability and other traits in some objective manner over time.

In the meantime, for our own little citizen-science experiment, I put the family on a high-fiber biota-building diet. I have no expectation that any amount of bran or chicory or artichoke will turn a reserved kid into an extrovert. The most cosmopolitan of gut microbiomes won't transform my elder daughter into the kid that waves her arms around to get a teacher's attention, nor is it going to put a perma-grin on her face. My goal is not to make her into a rowdy team player. That wouldn't be possible; it's not her.

But if having diverse gut microbiota is a nudge in the direction of lower social apprehensiveness or a heightened sense of social reward, then there's value. Heck, if a diverse microbiome has any positive effect at all on her health, resilience, and general oomph, it's worth it.

The goal is to eat as many different types of fiber as possible to shift the microbial diversity upward. I was amused to learn that each microbial species has its own tastes or fiber "preferences" depending on its genetic capacity to digest them. Offer a whole smorgasbord—millet and farro, chickpeas, Jerusalem artichokes, yams—and more species and subspecies of niche bacteria living low in the nooks and crannies of the gut lining will step up to the table. The more bacteria, the more different types of chemicals they'll exude, and the more synergy between them.

"Shoot for 30–40 servings of fiber a week," advises Leach, the notorious recipient of the Hadza fecal transplant. This translates into at least *twenty-five grams of fiber* daily. Leach is not just talking about sprinkling Metamucil on Cream of Wheat or stirring some powder into a strawberry smoothie. He means *a very large volume* of plants and resistant starches, although twenty-five grams is nowhere near the one hundred to one hundred fifty grams daily that modern hunter-gatherers eat. Twenty-five grams itself is a fantastical amount of fiber for most of us, especially my UJ, whose entire fiber reper-toire consists of oatmeal (loaded with milk and syrup) and bran flakes (sweetened). Like most American kids, she probably tucks in about eight grams of fiber on a good day. How are we going to reach twenty-five grams?

To eat all this grit, we need a game plan.

Biohack: The Fiber Points Game

Here's the way the game works. You need to get 25 grams of fiber from a variety of sources every day. The simplest way is to count the number of grams of fiber in a food. Each gram equals 1 Fiber Point. A banana has 3 grams of fiber in it, so if UJ eats it, she earns 3 Fiber Points; a slice of super-high-fiber whole-grain toast, 6 grams, so 6 Fiber Points. We find the number of grams on the sides of food containers or by looking them up on the Internet, and we tally them up on a whiteboard or in a notebook. Twenty-five Fiber Points a day. UJ haltingly dictates to the cellphone in kid robot voice. "How much fiber in one serving of spinach?" "How much fiber in one serving of chickpeas?" She looks at me slyly and puts the phone to her mouth. "How much fiber in milk chocolate?" I ask her to add it all up. For young kids, the Fiber Points Game doubles as an exercise in arithmetic.

There are three main classes of fiber that work in synergy with one another. Advanced players should aim to earn points in each category daily.

- *Soluble fibers* act as a prebiotic, feeding all the beneficial acid-making varieties of gut gatekeepers and immune stimulators. They dissolve in water and slow down the process of digestion so that microbes get their fill. Without soluble fiber, hungry microbes would gnaw away at the mucosal lining of the gut, triggering low-grade chronic inflammation. These special sugars also take up residence in the respiratory tract, where they block the attachment of disease-causing microbes. Sources include onions, peas, beans, greens, bananas, and many fruits. Hundreds of oligosaccharides are found naturally in breast milk and in Jerusalem artichokes, burdock, scallions, chicory, leeks, onions, and asparagus. Another form of soluble fiber is fructooligosaccharide, which is found in onions, chicory, garlic, asparagus, and bananas. Look for psyllium, too, which you can sprinkle on your oatmeal or spirit away into pancake batter. The more types of soluble fiber you can get your child to consume a week, the better.

Our family has developed an addiction to pudding made from chia seeds, which are exceptionally high in soluble fiber (11 grams per ounce). The basic recipe is simple enough for a child to make on her own: mix 3 cups of milk, ¾ cup of chia seeds, 2 tablespoons of maple syrup, and ½ teaspoon of vanilla in a large jar or bowl. Refrigerate for three or more hours. Enjoy. (Nut milks can be used in lieu of milk; add extra milk for a shake.)

- *Insoluble fibers* are in avocados, whole grains such as flaxseed and bran, and stringy veggie stalks. They speed up digestion and add bulk and sponginess to stool, but microbes can't ferment insoluble fibers as well as soluble fibers.

- *Resistant starches* are carbs, just not the (irresistible) ones in cake and bagels. They don't stick to the hips; instead, they go through the stomach and small intestine completely whole and undigested. Find resistant starches in seeds, raw oats that are bound within fibrous cell walls, yams, green bananas, and starchy white rice and potatoes that are cooked and cooled. Bifidobacteria and other major butyrate producers thrive on resistant starches, and many more thrive on the waste products of resistant-starch-eating bugs. We benefit immensely from this ecosystem.

Note that any given vegetable might contain several types of fiber: the potato, for instance, has a peel that has soluble fiber; cooling it produces resistant starch. The California Haas avocado has roughly a 60:40 ratio of insoluble-to-soluble fiber. Fibers work together in concert. Resistant starch works with bulky insoluble fiber to reach the bowel; otherwise it gets stuck in the upper colon, where it may cause harm.

Speaking of harm, different people react differently to the same foods depending on their existing baseline population of microbes in their gut and other factors. If not enough beneficial species are present, a high-fiber diet may lead to an imbalanced gut environment. To help avoid this, supplement with desirable species in yogurt, kefir, and other probiotic foods. As always, don't continue a diet if it doesn't feel right.

Diversity on the plate is diversity in the gut. One signal of adequate fiber is unambiguous: the stool itself. You know you're feeding the kid enough when he or she poops like a tribal child: large, soft, snakelike, two to three times a day. Before the Fiber Points Game, only the baby in our family could manage that.

"You're not eating fiber for *you.* You're certainly not eating fiber for *me.* You're eating it for your *good guys,*" I tell UJ. The appeal to the kid's generous heart and sense of higher self gets her to eat fiber-rich foods. She thinks of Lacts and Bifs as her pets, her superpowers. She shared my excitement when these guys proliferated last month, and she's motivated to keep them alive.

I admit, the concept of superhero microbes may not be altogether accurate (most aren't good or bad; it depends on context), but personifying them gets them well fed. Good guys mean a diverse population of mucin makers and fatty-acid producers. Good guys love avocado, whole wheat, celery, lentils. They covet the entire stalk of broccoli or asparagus, not just the pretty crown. They prefer pasta to have the flexibility of pipe cleaners, never mushy; their oatmeal steel cut, not instant; their carrots raw, not cooked. They like peas in brown rice with sesame seeds. A variety of tough seeds, shelled legumes, leathery root vegetables, stringy pods, and other tough plant matter provides a vast array of soluble fibers and resistant starches that bypass the stomach and arrive in the colon intact and ready for insatiable microbial marauders to ravish them. This is closer to the way humans ate in the past.

Hadza toddlers and kids eat as many as 150 grams of tough, gritty, molar-polishing fiber every day. If we in Western cultures could truly ever eat that much fiber, could we restore our ancestral microbiome to its full glory? Maybe, I wondered, if UJ could just eat a sufficient variety of fibers, invisible populations would rise out of her intestinal woodwork. Would that work?

Microbiologists Erica and Justin Sonnenburg addressed this question in their lab at Stanford University. First, they took a group of aseptically raised mice and colonized them with the gut bacteria of a human donor who had been raised on a high-fiber diet. That group represented our ancestral population. Then, half of those mice were randomly put on a low-fiber regimen for seven weeks. No surprise: the low-fiber group showed a serious decrease in gut microbiome diversity, with 60 percent of the species plummeting compared to the group who continued to eat high fiber. When the animals were put back on the high-fiber diet, *some but not all* gut microbe diversity was restored. Mice that had experienced the low-fiber lifestyle still had 33 percent less microbial diversity than the others.

Naturally, the Sonnenburgs were curious to see how much of the microbiome bounces back after *several* generations eat a low-fiber diet—not an abstract scenario if you think of our parents' and parents' parents' diets: shakes, puffs, canned spaghetti and meatballs, bologna on bread so white and refined you could squeeze it into a tiny ball. With every generation, it turned out, the babies of low-fiber eaters hosted fewer varieties of microbes compared to the babies of high-fiber eaters. By the fourth generation, the mice bred on low-fiber diets lost more than 70 percent of the microbial diversity of the original generation, especially from the Bacteroidales group of fiber-digesting butyric acid makers.

Now the big question: What happens when a line of low-fiber eaters goes back to a high-fiber diet? The Sonnenburgs switched the fourth-generation low-fiber pups to an "ancestral" high-fiber diet, and I was disappointed to learn that only *some* of the "good" species, but not all, rebounded. Their gut microbiome diversity was still 67 percent lower than that in mice whose family maintained a high-fiber diet. It seems that once some species are gone from the gut, they don't come back. They're gone forever. The only way to restore diversity, the Sonnenburgs found, was a fecal transplant from the mice with the high-fiber lineage, kind of like us getting a fecal transplant from the Hadza.

The Sonnenburgs' mice depressed me. It's a downer, this idea that even the grittiest high-fiber diet can't revive all species of bacteria once we wipe them out. But there's a difference between those mice and us. They live in a closed environment on a carefully controlled diet. We don't, and we can try to acquire (or reacquire) more microbes. The more variety of benign bacteria that we expose ourselves to via new (natural) foods and environments, the more potential we have for microbes to rebound or for a new species to pass through or even take residence for a while.

One way to do this is to eat a lot of foods that contain probiotics: yogurt, kefir, miso, kombucha, sauerkraut, sour cream, tempeh, pickles. This step may be a crucial one if you want to diversify your or your child's gut microbiome. The advice to eat a high-fiber diet to boost microbiome diversity assumes that there are enough "good guy" microbes already present in the gut. Problem is, many types of gut microbes feed on fiber, not only the "good guys," so in the absence of sufficient beneficial microbes, a high-fiber diet might drive an imbalance in the gut, and the diet would backfire terribly. Foods containing *Lactobacillus* and *Bifidobacteria* are recommended on a high-fiber diet (especially *L. rhamnosus* and *B. longum*, which are thought to be gentle enough for sensitive stomachs).

Remember, all these niche, diverse species we introduce to our guts have niche, diverse tastes. This is where all the *prebiotics* in the Fiber Points Game step up to the table: split peas, lima beans, artichokes, flaxseed, barley, avocados, figs, sundried tomatoes, and so on. So much is yet unknown about which species and strains are best, or best for us individually, so variety in the diet is the only way. See if you can get to one hundred different varieties. Switch things up.

The other major source of new microbes comes from the physical world around us. We don't live in an aseptic cage like the Sonnenburgs' mice. Everywhere, bacteria land on surfaces; some, encased in "resting spores," can survive for a long time before they find their way to our guts. People give off clouds of microbes. Some of the most common, *Lactobacillus* and *Bifidobacterium*, are shed from people, animals, and food into the environment and are found on surfaces and in dust, says James Scott, a microbiologist at the University of Toronto.

Consider, too, an emissary that delivers microbes directly to us: *Canis lupus familiaris*, the domesticated dog. A house where a dog lives contains more diverse microbes, including species of *Lactobacillus* that may be particularly protective against airway inflammation, decreasing the risk of allergies and asthma. Dogs share their gut bacteria with their humans.

Nature itself is full of microbes: they're in plants, in the soil, in the air. Most won't stick around in the gut, but while they're there or in our airways, they may influence mind and body. They can whisper to the vagus.

After all these efforts, how long does it take for a kid's gut microbiota to become more cosmopolitan? Our third round of gut microbe results (from uBiome) proves that it doesn't take much time. After a month of heavy yogurt consumption UJ's diversity percentile surged from the bottom quartile for an American (her first test the previous year) to *almost* average (second test). After two months of yogurt and one month of high Fiber Points, she went from almost average to slightly above average in diversity (third test). This suggests that she has successfully acquired more microbes in yogurt and other probiotics, and some stuck around. The more fibrous diet may have not only fed those good guys but also helped to revive tiny populations of other species that had lived in the nooks and crannies of her gut wall to the extent that they finally show up on a test. I'm not pretending that this level of gut biodiversity is anything close to our ancestral microbiome, but it's an improvement for sure.

It's a start, I tell her. Go, good guys!

Dogs are the magicians of the universe. —Clarissa Pinkola Estés

In any experiment, you look for results. After UJ's dramatic improvement in gut biodiversity, I ask myself if she has changed. She is certainly healthier than I expected for a winter month. With more diverse microbes in her gut, she's likely getting more nutritional value from food because each species has its ways to make more minerals bioavailable.

So, is she less anxious? Is she friendlier to strangers? Is she chattier? Is she embracing novelty better than ever before? Is she more "surgent"—or resourceful and emotionally responsive—as they'd say in a psychological profile? Better adjusted? I'm not expecting a social butterfly, but my maternal antenna tries to pick up on any subtle differences.

As in our Bifs and Lacts home experiment, or any self-test, you think you've seen evidence of change, then something happens that counters it, and it's unclear where it all balances out. You need studies with lots of people—the so-called big n—to be able to make any viable claims. Even if a diet has a positive outcome for many, it won't work for all; kids are individuals, starting from different starting points. In the future, we may have more targeted probiotic treatments based on genes and baseline gut microbe populations, and better ways to objectively track improvements. Now, all we can do is tinker and read the runes.

That said, one episode last week suggests a nudge in the right direction.

It was a cold afternoon; the kids and I were walking home from grocery shopping (chickpeas, barley, carrots, "ancient grains" mac and cheese). As we neared our building, we encountered an elderly man and a mutt that had a tail like a palm frond. Ami popped out of her stroller ("Dog! Dog!"), and the two girls rushed over, pulling off their mittens and offering their hands for a sniff. I let them proceed for a few minutes, then hauled the reluctant toddler and shopping bags up the stairs to our door. UJ stayed behind with the stroller and dog, and when I returned for the second trip, I was astonished. My reserved child had her hands all over the dog's muzzle. I saw its tongue lolling around, and all the while she was chatting up the owner. Their breath hung in the cold air, white puffs billowing in great breezy drifts. Was she was actually trying to charm him?

I had been talking about dogs recently. A dog, I'd said to UJ, does the dirty work of curating microbes for which we'd suffer a lot of indignity to acquire on our own. Had I planted the suggestion that dogs give us good microbes, which motivated her to start petting the dog, and then one thing led to another, which led to her chatting up a dog owner? Could I credit her extroverted mood that day to a better microbial toolkit, or, as before, to better health and nutrition, or was it nothing?

In any case, it was a beautiful moment that had to end. Ami was waiting in the foyer with her entire fist in her mouth, looking as if she might bolt.

UJ cast the dog owner a forlorn look. "Bye," she said, giving him a four-finger flutter and the dog a last pat.

"Such a friendly child!" the man said to me.

I laughed.

Once inside, she ran to the window, knocked on the glass, and then fluttered her hand some more.

It's as if in the dead of winter, she poked out of her cocoon.

MARCH

Let Them Eat Mudcakes

The psychological case for letting more outside in

S EVERAL YEARS AGO, at the Royal Marsden Hospital in London, an oncologist named Mary O'Brien noticed peculiar behavior in her patients with terminal lung cancer. She had inoculated them with *Mycobacterium vaccae* with the idea that the microbe might stimulate a faltering immune system. Weeks into the experiment, even as it became increasingly apparent that *M. vaccae* wasn't a cancer cure, O'Brien's treated patients started to feel clearer, happier, more alert, and more sociable. The study was double-blind; no one officially knew who was assigned the microbe or the placebo, but it was becoming clear which patients were treated with *M. vaccae*. If the microbe wasn't helping them physically, it sure seemed to help them cope mentally.

O'Brien knew that *M. vaccae* was in every sense a garden-variety microbe. Named after the cow in whose dung it was first discovered (*vacca* in Latin), *M. vaccae* is especially abundant in soil and grass-lands; it lives in crops and forests almost everywhere on the planet. *M. vaccae* can go airborne, which means that we inhale it when we're in earthy, leafy places. We ingest it too, in raw fruits and veggies. When we plunge our hands in dirt, *M. vaccae* may enter our bodies through little cracks in the skin. Back in the 1970s, scientists determined that inhaling, ingesting, and otherwise internalizing mycobacteria stimulates and trains the developing immune system to chill out and not to overreact to minor intruders. Kids growing up on farms or in rural areas don't suffer as much from asthma, allergies, hay fever, and other ailments as those growing up in urban areas do, thanks to early exposure to *M. vaccae* and other microbes.

Humans used to have constant contact with *M. vaccae*. It's what some microbiologists call an "old friend," but those days of intimacy are long gone as much of the world's population has moved away from its microbe-rich rural roots to a more hygienic urban and suburban life. Of course, we can't blame *M. vaccae* withdrawal for modern stress any more than the lack of fresh air, sun, relaxation, or community. But for the first time, O'Brien's finding prompted some scientists to think about the environmental microbiome beyond its role in allergy protection. Maybe our inner microbiome is much more connected with the outer one than we think, and *where* we are can affect our mental health, vis-à-vis microbes, as much as what we eat.

This isn't good news for most city kids. Like many, mine spend too much of their childhood indoors. Our outdoor experiences involve walking on concrete or asphalt, not soil. The air we breathe contains more exhaust than plant phytoncides. The kids' only association with dirt is the playground sandbox, which I banned after I kept finding grit in all the wrong places, like between the floorboards and bedsheets.

So, with *M. vaccae* on my mind and spring in the air, I resolve to spend more time in Central Park, perhaps the closest approximation to nature that a city kid can get. In early March there's more mud than grass there, but the children don't mind. Ami, now a one-year-old, has never walked on the bare earth before, and she takes to it like a wild animal freed from captivity. "Up, up, up!" she shrieks as she toddles up the hill, then down the hill, then up again, accelerating, zigzagging, belly out, bendy-kneed, strands of light downy hair aloft in the breeze. She is exuberant and raw, yet here I am, in panicked pursuit, to the smug amusement of dog walkers holding their charges on leashes. Unaccustomed to the uneven terrain, Ami eventually lands in mud and sludge. She stares at her dirty palms in happy disbelief. There is soil under her fingernails. There is bramble in her hair. And on her face there is a proverbial shit-eating grin.

That brown smear around her mouth? Evidence of primal contact with soil, just as I've been rooting for, clearly. I try to turn a gasp into a cheer.

Resilience is all about being able to overcome the unexpected.
—Jamais Cascio

Soon after Mary O'Brien published her cancer patient study in 2004, scientific interest in *M. vaccae* mushroomed. The microbe hadn't been known for stress resilience, but looking back it's no surprise. *Myco-bacterium* is distant kin of the soother *Bifidobacterium*; they're both members of the great phylum Actinobacteria, and both stimulate the human immune system. Many species of mycos exercise their powers in an unwelcome way—*Mycobacterium tuberculosis* and *Mycobac-terium leprae* (leprosy) come to mind, as well as milder pathogenic species in drinking water. But the myco named after the pastoral cow is associated with gentle immune stimulation.

One of the neuroscientists focused on *M. vaccae* was Christopher Lowry, then a researcher at the University of Bristol in England. Three times daily in a three-week experiment his team injected *M. vaccae* antigens into mice. They saw that the mice bodies started to pump out a higher-than-usual number of anti-inflammatory cytokines, the type that subdue an overactive immune response (the opposite of the inflammatory cytokines, which are triggered by infection). Later, when Lowry looked at the animals' brain tissue under a microscope, he saw that the anti-inflammatory cytokines had acted on sensory nerves that run to an area of the forebrain called the dorsal raphe nucleus, where you find serotonin-producing neurons. Lowry also saw that *M. vaccae* "selectively increased the density of microglia in the media prefrontal cortex," an area that communicates with the dorsal raphe nucleus and plays a leading role in fear expression. Observing the *M. vaccae* mice, Lowry saw that they were less afraid of their antagonist and less submissive generally. The *M. vaccae* seemed to offer at least three valuable benefits: first, to stimulate the production of soothing serotonin; second, to dial down stress-related anxiety in the prefrontal cortex; and third, to protect the brain from an overactive immune response to stress and the inflammation that follows.

What might all this mean in terms of behavior? A big clue lies in *M. vaccae*'s apparent ability to excite serotonin-releasing neurons. Serotonin is calming and an attention enhancer. If a kid needs to learn a tough new task or deal with a hard-nosed teacher, she'd do better with more serotonin in her system. Serotonin makes success more rewarding, so a student might stick to a task longer. Or he may cope with adversity better—when failing or being pushed—because his anxiety threshold will be higher, the same benefit we get from *Bifidobacterium* and *Lactobacillus*. Activation of serotonin neurons in the dorsal raphe region—the area that the *M. vaccae*-stimulated cytokines target—is linked with the ability to wait and be patient when there are delayed rewards. For children, this strength—as shown in the famous marshmallow test—is one of the earmarks of success later in life (see page 156). In other words, this little myco may indirectly enhance the capacity to be serene, persistent, and grounded. *Gritty.*

To test this hunch, Lowry, who is now at the University of Colorado at Boulder, subjected his mice to a variety of stressors. He tossed them in a bucket of water—the famed forced swim test—and saw how the *M. vaccae* mice swam with gusto, whereas more of the untreated mice went immobile. The serotonin sweet spot appeared to give them the spirit to keep kicking, just like mice inoculated with *Lactobacillus* in other research. When circumstances changed, they were calmer and more adaptable. Lowry's mice helped to explain why Mary O'Brien's lung cancer patients suddenly felt more life and fight even in their latest stages of the disease. Lowry called the *M. vaccae* effect "Prozac without the side effects." It appears to work as well as the drug.

After Lowry's initial discoveries biologists Dorothy Matthews and Susan Jenks at the Sage Colleges in New York took the experimentation a step further, seeing if *M. vaccae* improves how quickly mice learn and whether that knowledge would stick. The duo fed some of their mice *M. vaccae*–laced peanut butter and others regular chow, and then challenged them all to run through complicated mazes. The mycobacteria-fed mice not only learned the route twice as fast as the untreated ones, even as levels became increasingly complex, but also had twice the concentration and half the anxiety as those who weren't exposed.

The hypothesis behind Matthews and Jenks's experiment essentially boils down to this: Anxiety eats up cognitive bandwidth while serotonin increases motivation. *M. vaccae* simultaneously tamped down anxiety and increased motivation—a powerful double whammy. The remarkable mindset was observed in mice soon after they started the *M. vaccae* diet, as early as the first maze trial run, and tapered off about three weeks after they stopped eating the bacteria. But for the duration that *M. vaccae* stayed in their system, the rodents seem to have found that sweet spot we all seek for ourselves and our kids: to be both hyperfocused and ultrachill.

The connection between emotional resilience and *M. vaccae* is so fascinating that Lowry and his colleagues John Stanford (the first scientist to isolate the microbe in the 1970s) and Graham Rook tested it further. This time they introduced bullies into their experiment.

Think for a moment of childhood tormentors—the brutes or brats who snicker, push, and badmouth their peers with a sort of grinning scowl, breathing loudly through their nostrils. The rodent equivalent (usually a dominant male) causes other mice to flee in terror or to assume a submissive position called reactive coping. Lowry's mice had to deal with their bullies in their homes, nonstop, for nineteen days. But when the researchers injected some of the mice with a heat-treated *M. vaccae* vaccine three times over three weeks, the sufferers grew some backbone. Instead of bristling with anxiety and submitting as usual, they engaged in *proactive* coping, a term that has great appeal to parents. They stopped acting so meek and docile. They ignored their oppressor. They stopped trying to hide from him all the time. In a satisfying reversal, the *M. vaccae* mice, on occasion, would even attack and chase the tyrant around the cage.

The most amazing thing to me is the speed with which *M. vaccae* kicks in. The tables started to turn within the first hour of the experiment as the treated mice displayed fewer "flight" responses than their untreated peers. By the nineteenth day of the test period, about 70 percent of the *M. vaccae* mice displayed at least one proactive coping behavior, like outmaneuvering or striking back at the bully, compared to only 21 percent of the untreated mice. Even one to two weeks after their final dose of *M. vaccae*, the mice still had more spunk and fight in them than the untreated group, and they were more adventurous and exploratory once moved to separate housing.

In the animal experiments, subjects were injected with a heat-treated form of *M. vaccae*. In humans, it enters the body via natural routes. We inhale, eat, drink, or absorb the stuff. Lowry says that cells in the airways and gastrointestinal tract rapidly take up *M. vaccae* (and other microbes) and present them to the immune system (macrophage and dendritic cells). Once *M. vaccae*'s antigens and proteins bind to receptors on our immune cells, we ramp up production of regulatory T cells that suppress inflammation. The stress that comes from being pushed around and threatened normally kills off protective gut microbes, leading to a leaky gut, which then causes inflammation, which leads to greater anxiety. But *M. vaccae* may prevent inflammation, as it did in mice, resulting in a stable state of calm coping. Add to this the increased presence of soothing serotonin. When Lowry looked at the dorsal raphe in his subjects' brain tissue, he saw greater evidence of altered gene expression in serotonin-producing neurons compared to the control mice. This was a sign that serotonin was up.

Most recently, Lowry and colleagues with the Office of Naval Research found one more route by which *M. vaccae* increases stress resilience: sleep. Mice exposed to *M. vaccae* three times weekly slept more than a half hour longer on average each night than untreated mice, and their sleep was deeper. Surgically implanted brain wave recording devices showed that they spent more time in REM, the sleep mode that is essential to memory processing and stress coping. Can this help explain why UJ can't be roused from slumber and seems so "on" when we're in Vermont?

You, like me, might wish for a *M. vaccae* boost for yourself or your kids. Could this become what we've all been waiting for—a stress vaccine? A well-targeted serotonin blast and activation of an anti-inflammatory network could take the edge off any blade that life throws. As we know from Lowry's experiments, our immune systems respond to *M. vaccae* antigens and proteins. This means they work their magic even when the microbe is neither alive nor intact, which means it could, in theory, be packaged like other immunizations. Imagine the possibilities.

Anxious kids, public speakers, musicians, soldiers, anyone on edge would take that stress vaccine to cope with an anticipated stress. Within an hour or so it'd nudge them to a sweet spot during an exam, a performance, a trial, in battles big and small, in all the times that life feels like quicksand, and for all emotional ruts. More research is underway. In the meantime, we have dirt, leaves, forest air, unsprayed veggies, and mudcakes.

Biohack: Grounding

Our human ancestors encountered millions of *M. vaccae* and other microbes every day in mud and water. Were our forbearers better at coping with adversity for it? Nowadays, most of us probably encounter more people than *M. vaccae* in an average day, and that's a loss. Gardening is the obvious way to get exposure to beneficial soil bacteria, but it isn't the only route. Here are a few ways to increase your family's exposure to *M. vaccae* and/or other potentially beneficial plant and soil microbes:

- Put indoor plants in the kid's room. Plants fill a space with abundant and diverse microbes, not to mention help clean the air and potentially reduce reactive airways (from which city kids are especially prone to suffer). In one study, Austrian researchers put a few spider plants in a room and regularly swept the isolated space for microbes. Within six months the bacterial diversity on surfaces increased dramatically.
- Stop scrubbing the greengrocer or farmers' market produce (unless it has been sprayed with pesticides and fertilizers; always ask). Eat a hairy and hoary carrot raw; leave the beets unpeeled. *M. vaccae* are thought to be tenacious enough to resist light washing. Organic raw salad ingredients and uncooked veggies are likely to contain the microbe.
- "Forest bathe." The Japanese call it *shinrin-yoku*, the pastime of walking through a forest, breathing deeply, letting the microbes and other plant chemicals infuse the body for psychological health. Forest greenery is said to release phytoncides, which are airborne organic compounds with potential health-inducing properties.

- Encourage the kids to grow a garden, or just let them dig. This one's obvious, but when kids are in close contact with the earth, they'll breathe in M. vaccae and other soil and plant microbes, which are taken up by immune cells in the airways whereby they'll start to do their magic.
- Follow the ruminants. Grazing animals, like the cows for which M. vaccae is named, are in constant contact with the soil. M. vaccae lives on the udders of these animals, and contact with manure means contact with microbes, too. Children who live on farms early in life have a marked decrease in allergies and asthma.

A note of caution: Not all soil is safe. Don't let children eat food grown in or play on the dirt around old buildings, empty lots, construction sites, and even community gardens that may have been the location of an old structure. The risk is exposure to lead. Even at low levels in the blood (less than 5ppm), lead is a neurotoxin that harms children's brains. In short, it paralyzes new neurons, which changes the structure of the brain—and leads, irreversibly, to distractibility, lower IQs, and shorter attention spans. Although lead paint was banned in 1977 and lead gasoline in 1990, lead residue may still linger in the dirt that children can ingest or breathe in as easily as they do microbes.

Avoid, too, soil that's been recently sprayed with weed killers such as glyphosate (Roundup). Glyphosates are linked to much that can ail us: anxiety, depression, kidney and liver damage, allergies, asthma, celiac disease, birth defects, chronic fatigue, cancer, as well as genetic diseases and miscarriage—even autism. This is concerning, especially because glyphosates are detected in 93 percent of Americans' urine samples.

By midmonth I have a sense of what it's like to be a dog owner. The kids now want, *need*, to be walked in the park. Ami has learned to anticipate it. She puts on her coat and silver star shoes, then fetches my shoes and jacket for me and nudges me toward the door. Now! The leaves on the trees aren't out yet, but the grass has sprouted, and some days are hot in the way March never was in my childhood. I loiter, hands in pockets, with the other adults who've brought kids or dogs, as UJ and Ami do what comes to them naturally: they stomp in the mud, scratch at the dirt, snap dead twigs, hang on the low branches of a pine tree, pull weeds, spatter, and slather.

On one occasion Ami refuses to go back in her stroller at the appointed time. She arches her back and hollers. In a moment of clarity I see that the baby is taking away too much attention from UJ, and her demands are draining me.

"This Ami is too much," I say to UJ in mock seriousness. "Let's give this Ami away. But who'd take her?"

"I will," says UJ with certainty.

I continue, "What if I just trade her in for another Ami that's more reasonable and less demanding?"

"Mama!" She pauses for a moment, then says, "In my *Magic Tree House* book, Jack and Annie run into a piranha in the Amazon, and the piranha is really mean. But Mama, you can't blame the piranha. A piranha is what a piranha is. So, a baby is what a baby is. Ami is what Ami is. It's OK, Mama!"

Which of us is more grounded?

Measure what is measurable, and make measurable what is not so.
—Attributed to Galileo Galilei

When I ask researchers to quantify the *M. vaccae* exposure we'd need for noticeable results, I detect something like empathetic exasperation. We all want to know exactly how many airborne microbes we need to get anything like the coping skills of O'Brien's patients or Lowry's bully-resistant mice. But in the new psychobiology of bacteria, there's so much we don't know, can't tell, can't calculate.

Lowry's current research, he says, will determine how much concentration of *M. vaccae* dispersed in the air is enough to confer health benefits in mice—information that will get us one step closer to knowing how much humans need to breathe in for it to have a behavioral effect on us. (In the meantime, *M. vaccae* capsules are available online for experimental use, but they're expensive and may not be as effective.) After the mice studies, more research on humans will follow. It's just another instance of public (and parental) curiosity outpacing the scientific process.

The funny thing, Lowry admits, is that maybe there's nothing all that special about *M. vaccae* except its presence just about everywhere on the planet and the fact that it has been coexisting with our species since time immemorial. He believes that there are hundreds, maybe thousands of other microbes in our natural environment that also have transformative effects on our behavior and immune systems, especially others in the phylum Actinobacteria.

Another promising environmental microbe is *Clostridium butyricum* (a member of the phylum Firmicutes), which, like *M. vaccae*, is found in soil all around the world. Not long ago, a research group in China fed *C. butyricum* to mice with vascular dementia, a condition in which memory and learning are hobbled. The treated mice learned to escape mazes faster, and their spatial skills were superior to their untreated peers with the same condition.

When the researchers euthanized the *C. butyricum*–enriched fast learners and looked at thin slices of their brain tissue, including the hippocampus, which forms and stores memory, they saw striking differences from the others. The *C. butyricum* group had higher levels of brain-derived neural growth factor, BDNF, which acts like fertilizer for new neurons. Like *Bifidobacterium*, it's thought that these microbes increase signaling up the vagus nerve, which in turn stimulates growth factors in the brain. (Note that other members of *Clostridia*, such as *C. difficile* and *C. botulinim*, are extremely detrimental to us and release toxins that also talk to the brain via the vagus nerve.)

It may be important to mention that the *C. butyricum*–dosed mice had higher levels of—no surprise—butyrate in their stool samples. This fatty acid, which some species of *Clostridium* are so good at churning out in our guts, feeds many other types of healthy bacteria, especially *Lactobacillus*, and supports uncommon species. Is it a coincidence that the fastest, nimblest learners in the study also had higher gut microbe diversity?

It is apparent that no lifetime is long enough in which to explore the resources of a few square yards of ground. —Alice M. Coats

Let's face it, an urban green space is to the wilderness what a dread-locked hipster is to a hunter-gatherer. After a while, I started to get suspicious of the so-called urban soil microbiome. Urban soil is bombarded by air pollution, pesticides, fertilizers, and untold other toxic assaults. I began to doubt that Central Park would harbor *M. vaccae*. It seemed to me that the city soil would have much less microbial diversity compared to the dirt in rural Vermont, where we spend our summer holidays, and that the Vermont soil microbiota would be less diverse than that in purer, wilder places like the Himalayas or the Honduran rainforest.

Adding to my skepticism was the sign that UJ saw taped to a London plane tree near the entrance to the park's playground. The print was small and almost illegible, but we understood it to say that the grass had been treated with glyphosate, a potent broad-spectrum herbicide. Glyphosate, the generic name for Roundup, is sprayed three thousand times a year in urban green spaces in New York City and on crops everywhere. It's the most widely used agricultural chemical in the world, although several countries have banned it.

I tell UJ that the spray kills weeds.

"What's wrong with weeds?" UJ asks innocently. "Does this mean the park's not natural?"

"Well. It's an evergreen topic, the debate over what's 'natural,' isn't it?" I say.

That gives her pause.

A city park is certainly less "natural" than an unmaintained forest, and after the glyphosate warning I had even less conviction about the nature of urban soil. So, I turned to ecologist Kelly Ramirez, who studies soil microbiome in areas around the world, including urban soil, and happens to have studied New York City's Central Park in particular. A couple years ago, when Ramirez was a postdoc researcher at Colorado State University, she and her team collected nearly six hundred soil samples throughout the park, sequenced the microbiota, and then compared the results to those from tropical forests, grasslands, tundra, and deserts around the world. And what did they find? A wasteland dominated by only the toughest, most aggressive microbes? A sad, scrappy ghost of what was once the multitudinous microbiome of Manahattan?

No. To everyone's amazement, the urban soil was as diverse as the legendary American melting pot. The lab results showed no difference at all between the magnitude of soil microbes in the Central Park dirt compared to those found in some of the wildest and remotest places on Earth. This was incredible to me. In a teaspoon of soil you'll find about one billion bacteria. Of the nearly 2,500 phylotypes of common bacteria in worldwide samples, Central Park's shared an unimaginable 94.7 percent overlap. Ramirez and team found a mind-boggling 167,000 species of bacteria, archaea, and eukaryotes. That's an awesome amount of biodiversity, right here in a place you'd think of as almost completely artificial. Microbes have survived and made it here like any other New Yorker! Of note, more than 1 percent of the microbes cataloged were urban exotics that were only found in Central Park and nowhere else on Earth.

Ramirez told me that mycobacteria are certainly present in Central Park, and that the species *M. vaccae* is quite common generally, although her study didn't drill down to species level. If you look at her data for Actinobacteria, the phylum that includes *Mycobacterium* and *Bifidobacterium* as well as hundreds of other organisms that may be similarly promising for mental health, you'd be shocked. The study found a greater abundance of Actinobacteria in our urban jungle than in global soils in general.

There's a rule of thumb when evaluating any piece of land for soil microbes: the more diversity of plants you see growing above the soil, the more microbial diversity below. Central Park has diversity built into its design, with a variety of botanical habitats including wooded areas, ponds, fields, and gardens that are home to 174 different species of trees in the park. No one sees the soil microbes, but they're the foundation of it all.

When I asked Ramirez about the glyphosate sprayings in the park, she said that herbicides are not a threat to the soil microbiome when applied sparingly, and it certainly appears that the park hadn't been sprayed heavily in the places tested. Other research, however, offers damning evidence that the chemical kills soil microbes, especially after multiple applications, and can wipe out gut bacteria, too. In our intestines, microbes like *Lactobacillus* begin to break down the glyphosates—another gift to us—but the toxin leaves them significantly weakened. Lactobacilli then produce fewer healthy amino acids than usual, and glyphosate-resistant pathogens such as *Clostridium difficile* and *Salmonella* species are likelier to take over the gut. Ominously, one of the amino acids harmed by glyphosate is tryptophan, the precursor of serotonin.

There is no evidence that the amount of glyphosate we're normally exposed to in food or at a park harms our gut microbiota significantly. But there's also an absence of research: in vitro studies on people— especially dirt-eating children—have yet to be done, and it's tough to disentangle the effects of just one chemical on the whole microbiome. There is a very real concern that this herbicide alters the types of microbes that can thrive on the leaves and stems of the plants we eat, if not the ones in the soil itself. Only the microbes that are most resistant to the herbicide would be in our food—and "good guys" like *M. vaccae* might not be among the lucky survivors.

If you don't like bacteria, you're on the wrong planet.
—Stewart Brand

After multiple, frequent exposures to mud and greenery, I expected the kids to be teeming with *M. vaccae*. But if you look for *Mycobacterium* in a standard gut microbiome test, as I did, you won't find them. There's no easy, effective way to measure these guys in us. It's hard to dose these microbes in a bite or an inhale, and there's no record of which plants exude the most of these microbes, under which conditions.

But just because there's no easy way to measure *M. vaccae* in us doesn't mean that they aren't there. They do survive in the gut, Lowry explains, but not in numbers like *Lactobacillus* or *Bifidobacterium*; there's not enough to pass the filters on tests. Another obstacle in detecting *M. vaccae* involves their structure: they have cell walls that are hard to break down, and require more complex DNA extraction than do other microbes. This gives them a shadowy reputation for being "hidden" in healthy people.

This is where you *will* find mycobacteria: the oral microbiome. It's in the upper airways, the nostrils, and the inside of the cheeks. We inhale these buggers even more often than we ingest them. Lowry explains that rapidly, within hours, *M. vaccae* are taken up into the body by a special messenger in the mucus, the microfold (M) cells, which deliver the microbe to the immune system, which in turn translates messages into anti-inflammatory cytokines and serotonin surges. *M. vaccae* use different pathways from gut bacteria, but they're just as effective and efficient. This may explain why *M. vaccae*–exposed mice develop an uncanny ability to cope with stressors within hours of exposure, whereas gut microbes may take longer to influence our behavior.

This may also help explain why, after an afternoon in green space, a kind of radiance can come off the kids. Even today, on a blustery after-school stroll in late March, their dirty faces shine.

Sadly, the spell fades a bit the moment we step outside the gate and a dark cloud of exhaust descends on us. UJ stops. Her face takes on an inscrutable expression, suggesting absorption with the spectacle of people eating hot dogs, chicken biryani, and cola. "Disgusting!" she proclaims, making a big show of fanning the air and wrinkling her nose. She points to the food cart's gasoline-powered generator. "Stop polluting!" she shouts at the vendor and gives him a menacing stare. Who'd guess that this is a kid who can be too shy to ask the waitress at the diner for another pancake? The man scowls, and I worry that he'll lash out. As the smoky haze settles into the park's greenery, I grab my daughter's hand and hustle her away.

This is what I tell myself: if all those microbes can make it here, they can make it anywhere. With the right boosts, maybe we can too.

II

Outside/In

———

APRIL

The Stardust in Us

An essential mineral has been lacking in our diets for generations. What happens when we bring it back?

ONCE UPON A time, carrots were so healthy that you had to eat only one to get the same amount of nutrients in three carrots today. For every three bites of broccoli our kids eat, my generation (growing up in the 1980s) needed only two to get the same quantity of several minerals. Our children must eat nearly twice as many potatoes to get as much iron as their grandparents or great-grandparents did in the 1940s, and the same goes for spinach and grains. Magnesium intake has declined by half, even among people who eat their veggies.

Comparing nutrient concentrations in food crops today with those from a half century ago, the University of Texas biochemist Donald Davis found 43 percent less iron, 19 percent less calcium, and 38 percent less B2 (riboflavin). Davis says there have almost certainly been declines in other nutrients not routinely measured back then: zinc, vitamins B6 and E, sulfur, selenium, copper, dietary fiber—and magnesium. Trace minerals have become shadows of themselves.

"That's not fair!" UJ protests before I go further. What I'm telling her is the very opposite of the classic walk-to-school-in-the-snow stories to make children feel grateful that they don't have it as bad as their forebears. This story makes her indignant. She feels cheated. She must work harder—shovel in two or three times as much spinach and cabbage and tomatoes and cauliflower—to get the same nutritional benefit her grandparents did from eating older varieties of these same fruits and veggies, and even more so compared to our ancestors who ate the plants' wilder predecessors. (I don't tell her that modern fruits and veggies are also arguably less flavorful than those in Grandma's time.) Where did all the missing minerals go?

Davis points to the dark underbelly of the green revolution, which began more than fifty years ago. To feed the world's booming population, agronomists developed crops that were faster-growing and more pest-resistant than ever before. But the new varieties are nutritional weaklings: they can't produce or suck up enough nutrients from the soil to keep up with their Jack-and-the-Beanstalk rate of growth.

The broccoli that great-grandma cooked might have been looser and sparser with a more flowery head, but it was packed with more nutrients than the tightly clustered variety grown today. Whatever nutrients are in many modern fruits and veggies are further diminished through premature picking, handling, refrigeration, transport, and storage.

As if this weren't bad enough, recent studies show that nutrient drain is worsening due to climate change. Rising levels of carbon dioxide make plants even faster-growing, higher-yielding, and more carbohydrate heavy, at least in the short term. But again, accelerated growth reduces micronutrients. Studies on major crops such as rice and wheat, lettuce and spinach show that elevated CO_2 leads to less protein, nitrogen, phosphorus, potassium, sulfur, zinc, copper, and magnesium (which was about 25 percent lower than the control condition in a study at Kansas State University).

Then, to make the matter worse (literally) are the missing soil microbes. As carbon dioxide increases in the atmosphere, some scientists are pinning their hopes on soil microbes, which increase under high CO_2 conditions and help nourish plants. But what's happening to the microbes in the soil where our food is grown?

"Microbes!" UJ cries, rolling her eyes to the ceiling. She's starting to get the sense that everything in the world comes down to microbes.

Normally, a plant has a whole community of soil microbes that live around it, called the rhizosphere. The rhizosphere exists because the plant chugs out carbs that microbes love, called exudates. In return, microbes break down minerals—magnesium, calcium, molybdenum, and others—in the soil to make them more bioavailable to the plant, and then shepherd those by-products directly to the plant's roots. It's a happy, symbiotic relationship. But—here's the problem—if a plant is sprayed with glyphosates and fed fertilizers, as most are, it becomes lazy. It stops feeding the soil microbes. Then there are no more microbes.

A bell pepper plant or a grapevine does not know that by welching on this ancient trade with microbes it's missing out on micronutrients that nourish its growth and protect its roots from oxidative stress. Magnesium is the central atom in the chlorophyll molecule, and without it plants can't capture the sun's energy. Magnesium powers photosynthesis. Even if a farmer sprays extra magnesium, iron, and other nutrients into the soil, those minerals aren't as bioavailable to the plant as they would be had microbes been there to help the plant absorb them. If the farmer also sprays with the herbicide glyphosate—again, most do—the chemical binds with nutrients so that even fewer are available to the plant. The plant is less nourished, and so is the plant eater.

UJ squints at her heaping plate of kale. She measures her words carefully. "How many bites do I need to eat tonight?"

The body needs four major minerals: magnesium, calcium, potassium, and sodium. Of the four, magnesium is the one most frequently missing from the modern diet. Most kids are growing up without even half the magnesium that their grandparents and older generations took in. At least 75 percent of us are deficient in this mineral, and we don't even know it.

Problem is, if this generation's fruits and veggies have less magnesium and other nutrients than did past varieties, few kids are compelled to compensate by eating more. At the supermarket at this time of year, my girls find mangos that could double as Paleolithic hand axes, pellet-like berries, bland bananas (no appeal), a honeydew melon so pale it looks as if it were grown in a crypt, and tomatoes that manage to look both tough skinned and anemic.

How can we make up for our major mineral deficits?

We are stardust, we are golden, we are billion-year-old carbon, and we've got to get ourselves back to the garden. —Joni Mitchell

You might say there are two trends going in opposite directions. The farm-raised fruits and veggies are getting lazier and slacking off, while the children are arguably working harder and are more stressed out. The American Psychological Association's Stress in America survey reported some troubling statistics to chew on. Children ages eight to seventeen are more worried than previous generations had been about doing well in school, getting into good colleges, and their family's finances. About one in three get headaches regularly. Nearly 45 percent of kids in that age group also reported having sleeping difficulties. Perhaps most worrying, only a small percentage of parents knew or could tell that their kids were stressed.

A mineral-poor diet contributes to stress. Or, let me put it another way: a mineral-poor diet offers no stress buffer. And as it turns out, magnesium, the mineral that's most depleted in modern crops, is the one that may de-stress and improve sleep.

A quick refresher on magnesium. Magnesium is one of the most abundant elements in the universe, born of the thermal fusion of helium and neon. The magnesium here on Earth once piggybacked on the meteorites that formed the early Earth—it's stardust. Magnesium is in our planet's crust, its mantle. It's in the seawater. It's in every type of cell in every type of organism. It's in the chlorophyll heart of plant cells. The stardust is in us. Just not as much as it used to be, or needs to be.

Now, if kids didn't have *any* magnesium they wouldn't grow. Without a tiny but crucial quantity, their hearts wouldn't beat. Their bones and teeth would crumble: magnesium fortifies the lattices on which calcium is deposited. Their blood wouldn't clot, their muscles and neurons wouldn't work, they wouldn't be able to regulate their body temperature or any of the other 296 biochemical reactions in the body for which magnesium is required. Most kids are fine when it comes to beating hearts, breathing, moving, staying warm.

It's the higher-level functionality where a deficiency might show up, and the more deficient, the more severe the symptoms. Without enough of the old stardust, children get spacier: the synaptic connections between neurons weaken, which in turn weakens memory and learning ability. They get brain fog. The worse their deficiency, the harder it is for them to organize their thoughts or maintain a conversation without trailing off. *Ummmm.* Low-mag people complain of headaches, lack of concentration, nervousness, tingling feet, cramps in the soles of the feet and toes and neck. Kids are agitated easily and won't sleep as well or as long. They're likelier to get overwhelmed. It's all part and parcel.

The test of all knowledge is experiment. —Ralph Waldo Emerson

My children are not just guinea pigs this month. They'll be magpies, selectively seeking a certain shiny, silvery metal. Their magnesium levels will be increased, topped off, and then we will see if there's any shift in their mood or behavior. That's the experiment.

Starting out, I know for sure that my elder daughter comes nowhere near the recommended daily allowance of 130 milligrams a day of magnesium on her chosen diet of bread, butter, oatmeal, parmesan cheese, and pancakes. (That's a minimum; some authorities call for five times one's weight in milligrams.) Although a cup of cultured yogurt offers up to 30 milligrams, and we've had a lot of yogurt so far this year, I'm not sure that cuts it.

For a six-year-old to reach that daily target 130 milligrams of magnesium, she'd have to eat four bananas a day or two servings of black beans or five tablespoons of peanut butter. She could theoretically get enough magnesium in fewer than three cereal bowls' worth of oat bran, but magnesium in grains is less easily absorbed by the body. Green leafy vegetables are the best bet: one cup of spinach or chard—cooked, boiled, drained, salted or not—reaches the daily target.

Four bananas. One cup of spinach. How hard is this?

Easy peasy on a one-off basis. (About two and a half cups of peas also fulfill the quota.) Fortunately for us, we've been on a fiber-heavy diet for a month now, and high-fiber foods often have a fair amount of magnesium. This month, I start thinking of our dinners through the filter of magnesium: what foods are highest in it? We mix and match lentils with kale and a handful of cashews. Spinach is a high-mag shortcut, so I throw more into a sauce. I triple the recipe for my high-mag chickpea soup with kale and couscous and make the kids eat it for both snack and dinner. I learn that a plate of kale freshly picked and driven in from upstate that morning likely has more magnesium than the kale that took the multiday voyage from faraway farmland to big box supermarket, so I look for foods grown locally. (See the box on page 84 for foods with highest magnesium values.)

It's not always easy. We're swimming against the current in some ways. Our ancestors used to top up on magnesium simply by drinking water from mineral-rich streams and lakes, but magnesium is often filtered out of municipally treated water, and if it isn't, it's treated with fluoride, which binds to magnesium and makes it unavailable to the body. We Westerners love our cheese and milk and yogurt, but the calcium in those foods competes with and prevents us from absorbing magnesium. We need magnesium to synthesize glucose (a mag deficiency is linked with type 2 diabetes), but our high-sugar diet, too, depletes magnesium.

There are two reasons why I decided to give the children an occasional magnesium supplement on top of our increasingly healthy diet. First, some researchers suggest that kids should take *more* than the daily allowance to achieve the best antianxiety results, so I want to make sure that we have a sufficient amount (for scientific purposes, of course). Second, we're trying to dig ourselves out of the hole of a long-term deficit. It may take all month, or several months, of increased magnesium consumption to recoup our losses.

For the young child who doesn't eat her veggies, insurance comes in the form of a magnesium lotion, Epsom salts, pills, powders, or sprays (again, see text box for details). A supplement of one hundred milligrams of magnesium, the minimum used in studies, is considered a modest and harmless boost. A potentially easier route than the alimentary canal is a transdermal one, through the skin. Researchers in the United Kingdom found that a spray of 31 percent magnesium chloride raises cellular magnesium levels by 60 percent over three months, although it must be said that the study was funded by an herbal research center rather than an academic lab. (Why science has never embarked on a simple gold-standard controlled study of transdermal magnesium absorption, I cannot say, except to speculate that the mineral is so plentiful that it's not profitable. It's, well, dirt cheap.)

Magnesium spray can sting, so it's best applied to the sole of a child's foot where the skin is tougher. This calls for a spritz and a foot massage, which is what I find myself giving the kids five minutes before lights out. Luckily, they love the ritual. For once, UJ is not tussling or squirming. Little Ami picks up the bottle with great enthusiasm and pretends to spray and rub her big sister's foot and then her own. Five sprays on each sole, ten sprays in total, amount to about 130 milligrams of magnesium. Easy. UJ lays on her faux silk pillow, her golden-brown hair splayed out around her, eyes closed. Wooziness falls over us, and even the bedside light seems somehow dimmer. It happens that magnesium sulfate is used to quiet down or "dope" racehorses.

Get yourself grounded and you can navigate even the stormiest roads in peace. —Steve Goodier

If you're going to megadose on magnesium like us (or even aspire to reach the minimum), you probably want scientific proof that you're doing the right and salutary thing. What's so bad about being magnesium deficient, anyway? Most of us are, and we get by, right?

We need more research, as many studies aren't large or well controlled. But what science knows for sure is that even minor magnesium deficiencies are linked with subtle but undesirable mental health consequences. Magnesium-deficient people report feeling more anxious, depressed, and apprehensive than those with normal levels; once their levels rise, they feel more grounded. An analysis of over five thousand participants in the National Health and Nutrition Examination Survey found that people who fall short of the recommended daily intake of magnesium have higher levels of inflammation and C-reactive protein, a biomarker of stress.

Among children, magnesium deficiency has overlapped with hallmark signs of attention deficit hyperactivity disorder (ADHD): inattention, lack of focus, and a tendency to make hasty, poor choices without considering long-term consequences. An Egyptian study found that when six- to sixteen-year-old kids with attention deficit disorder were supplemented with two hundred milligrams of magnesium per day for eight weeks, their attention skills improved, at least going by their parents' ratings. Moms and dads noted that their kids' impulsivity and hyperactivity lessened, along with (I take note) oppositional attitudes, while an untreated control group showed no improvement. (More magnesium, less mouthiness?) A similar trial, also small, came to the same conclusion, and in its follow-up noted that when kids stopped taking the magnesium supplement, they defaulted to their previous inattentive and hyperactive state within weeks. (Again, I take note.)

To understand how magnesium reduces the stress response, you need to first consider the body's HPA axis (hypothalamic-pituitary-adrenal). When we're pressured, the hypothalamus (H) in the brain responds by releasing a siren cry called corticotropin-releasing hormone. This signal reaches the pituitary (P) gland, located underneath the brain, which in turn responds by triggering production of ACTH (adrenocorticotropic hormone). *Stress!* (A low-magnesium diet is often linked with higher ACTH.) The adrenal (A) glands above the kidneys pick up on the slightest whiff of ACTH in the bloodstream and respond by releasing the stress (fight-or-flight) hormone cortisol, which gets past the blood-brain barrier.

Cortisol helps us spring to action, and it's the right fuel for running from an attacker or thinking on one's feet. But *chronic* cortisol exposure—a steady stress drip—leads to not only anxiety and jitteriness but also inflammation, weaker immunity, and weight gain. Once too much cortisol reaches the brain it impairs the hippocampus and prefrontal cortex, leading to a loss of neurons and then fuzzy or scattered thinking, depression, memory loss, and learning impairments.

Too much cortisol, and we stop thinking intently, flexibly, creatively, or rationally. Trying to plan and organize in this state is like trying to read while screaming. Cortisol also stimulates the amygdala, the area of the brain that calls up feelings of panic, fear, and anxiety. The fateful result: the hypothalamus releases yet more cortisol, the stress cycle burns on, and the child burns out.

Except when magnesium stops the cycle, and this is where it plays a starring role. Magnesium has a surprising influence over the pituitary gland, which sits right outside the blood-brain barrier. It can dial down the pituitary's production of ACTH early on in the stress cycle. Without as much ACTH in circulation, the adrenals downstream don't get the distress signal that tells them to pump out so much cortisol. Anxiety averted. The stress hormonal system is balanced, including the thyroid and sex hormones, which leads to mental balance. A kid can relax and grow.

Magnesium also plays a role inside the brain, although the forms that we usually ingest or spray on our skin don't pass through the blood-brain barrier easily. (Magnesium threonate, a synthesized form taken in pill form, is a recent exception.) Nevertheless, enough magnesium must enter to do its crucial work of protecting a type of receptor called NMDA (N-methyl-D-aspartate) which controls synaptic plasticity, the ability of synapses to strengthen or weaken when remembering new facts and skills. Without enough magnesium to guard the vulnerable open channels of the NMDA receptors, they become overactivated, a state that's toxic to nerve cells. You don't want this for yourself or your children. An overactive NMDA receptor leads to reduced BDNF ("brain fertilizer," see page 63), anxiety, forgetfulness, brain fog, and, over time, damaged neurons.

Any parent who has seen a darling child melt down on the sidewalk knows that once the stress cycle starts, it's hard to stop. The cruelest part is that stress drains the body of magnesium, perpetuating the stress cycle and the downward spiral. If children are magnesium-deficient *before* getting stressed—and so many are—the stress exacerbates the deficiency. It's as if in the crash and burnout they also lose their brakes and suspension. Chronic magnesium deficiency is also linked with apathy, irritability, and restlessness—all related to stress. Magnesium-deficient kids are sulkier.

I'm sold.

The mineral world is a much more supple and mobile world
than could be imagined by the science of the ancients.
—Pierre Teilhard de Chardin

"Hey, Mama," UJ says, giving me one of her sly smiles over a thirty-milligram-of-magnesium serving of broccoli rabe. ("The bitterer the better," she says, just to be provocative.) "Is the magnesium feeding the good guys?" She's thinking about her beneficial gut microbes. All those sanctimonious talks left her with an impression that gut bacteria are lurking in everything.

Turns out, the comparison between the gut and the soil is apt. Both are at their best when bursting with diverse microbes. Microbes in the soil transform, break down, and deliver magnesium for plants, and microbes in our gut do the same for us. As an example of how much we need microbes to absorb magnesium (and other minerals), look at whole grains. Magnesium binds to the fiber and phytates in these gristly grains, and our own gut enzymes can't break it down well enough to release it. As smug and virtuous as we are about feeding our kids eight-grain sprouted wheat bread and bulgar-freekah patties, all that deliciousness won't do them much good unless they can absorb the nutrients. A kid who has a lot of diverse microbial fermenters is going to get a lot more magnesium from that meal.

Studying a strain of *B. bifidum* in an in vitro experiment, Polish researchers discovered that the more of it present in the gut, the more magnesium was released from food (along with zinc, manganese, and copper). In another experiment, rats were fed fructooligosaccharides that are digestible only to microbes—especially *Bifidobacterium* and *Lactobacillus*—and, as a result, the animals' magnesium (and iron) levels soared. The microbe-magnesium relationship goes both ways. When mice are magnesium-deficient, their population of calm-inducing microbes nosedives. The mice get depressed and anxious.

Eat all your broccoli rabe, UJ, and you'll get kefir for dessert.

Biohack: Calming Down to Earth

In any household with children, chances are one of the following challenges presents itself at any given time: trouble falling asleep, performance stress, anxiety, depression, and deep undercurrents of worry (and we're not just talking about the parents). If any of these issues apply, consider magnesium, short- or long-term, as a gentle therapy. Most adults are magnesium deficient, and so are most kids, especially kids who eat few veggies and a lot of cheese and milk (which reduce magnesium absorption). The less microbiota diversity and population of bacterial fermenters in the gut, the harder it is to extract magnesium and other nutrients from food.

A deficiency doesn't show up on a normal blood test. Ninety-nine percent of the body's supply of magnesium is stored in bone, muscle, the brain, and soft tissue—not exactly easy places to access. Some medical researchers recommend the Magnesium RBC essential mineral test, which measures the tiny amount of magnesium in red blood cells. This test and another that measures ionized magnesium are the two used in the research studies. The RBC test can be ordered online without a prescription.

Per the National Institutes of Health, the recommended daily intake of magnesium for children ages one to three is 80 mg, ages four to eight is 130 mg, ages nine to thirteen is 240 mg, and ages fourteen to eighteen is 410 mg for males and 360 mg for females. (However, some nutritionists say that an optimal dose is about five times a person's body weight in milligrams of magnesium, so a 50 pound kid would get 250 mg.) It may take weeks or months to recover from a deficiency.

How to get the conservative daily quantity of 130 milligrams of magnesium into a small child?

- Supplement. The element is unstable in its pure state, so supplements can be taken in many compound forms: magnesium oxide (which has limited bioavailability and may take up to a month to restore levels), magnesium citrate (a powder that can loosen the bowels too much, causing an unpleasant bathroom experience especially unsuited to kids), or magnesium sulphate (Epsom salt in a bathtub). Or—perhaps the best bet for children—magnesium chloride, an oil that feels a bit like heavy saltwater. As a spray, it's best tolerated when diluted or in gel form, applied to the soles of the feet. I can rub several sprays into my daughter's foot without protest. My tough-soled toddler loves it.

- Real food. Supplements are no substitute for real food. The under-eight set need at least 130 "Magnesium Points" a day, which can— yes, really—be achieved with veggies. Even though we're no longer eating our grandma's super spinach, the stuff at the grocery store still has antioxidants, phytonutrients, vitamins, and other minerals that growing kids can't get elsewhere, and we need other vitamins and minerals, such as B6 and boron, to keep magnesium inside the cells. Importantly, whole foods also have calcium, which stays in balance with magnesium. Chances are, if a kid has scored his 25 Fiber Points a day, he's also earned enough magnesium as a bonus. (In our family, chia pudding gives us a mag fix as well as high fiber points.) Here's a quick point sheet with prime sources:

1 oz pumpkin seeds	74 mg	1 cup cooked spinach	157 mg	¼ cup seaweed (kelp)	24 mg
1 oz dark chocolate	41 mg	1 cup Swiss chard	29 mg	20 cooked clams	34 mg
½ cup almonds	191 mg	1 cup kale	31 mg	½ cup tofu	37 mg
½ cup cashews	200 mg	1 cup collards	10 mg	1 cup cooked lentils	71 mg
¼ cup pistachios	37 mg	½ cup mustard greens	9 mg	½ cup lima beans	40 mg
1 cup buckwheat	393 mg	½ cup dried apricots	21 mg	1 oz chia seeds	95 mg
1 cup brown wild rice	84 mg	1 banana	32 mg		
1 cup oatmeal	61 mg	½ cup dried figs	50 mg		

If you, like me, have wondered if organic fruits and veggies have more magnesium than nonorganic, here's the upshot. It depends on the maturity of the farm where the food is grown. The longer the soil has been cultivated using organic methods, the more minerals can enrich the soil, and the more the soil microbes can flourish. A newly converted organic farm, however, may be no better in this regard than the nonorganic one it had recently been. Unless you know the farmer or grow the plant yourself, you don't know for sure if it has more minerals. (Some of us, however, insist that you can often tell by the flavor.)

That said, some organically grown produce has 30 percent higher levels of antioxidants and other phytochemicals (including immune-boosting polyphenols, flavonols) than conventionally grown equivalents. Organically grown crops need to develop these compounds as self-defense mechanisms (against sunlight, insects, bacteria, and fungi), while lazy pesticide-sprayed plants do not. These substances are often antioxidants, and they protect our cells, too.

There is a time for many words, and there is also a time for sleep.
—Homer

I cannot say whether the children's baseline anxiety is lower than usual in the magnesium weeks, but there is a benefit I see immediately, night after night, and it's linked with lower anxiety and just as precious: an easier time falling asleep. Calm before sleep. More solid sleep. Bedtime has taken the air of fairyland intimacies, the atmosphere heavy. The oil leaves a slight residue on my child's sole, as if she had just been out at sea and went ashore to sleep under the stars.

Yes, after four weeks of magnesium nearly every night, I can say, hand on heart, that my children generally sleep longer and more soundly. There was the Sunday morning that UJ didn't emerge from her bedroom until ten o'clock, blinking like a newborn baby. If a day has been particularly emotional or overstimulating, a few squirts of magnesium spray seems to help both children fall asleep quickly. Maybe it's the ritual foot massage that ushers them to sleep, but something is working. (A handful of pumpkin seeds or a bedtime banana might do the trick, too.) It often, but not always, offsets my insomnia. (It's best for mild cases.)

There is increasing scientific support for the observation that magnesium ushers in deep sleep faster. More than three decades ago,

German scientists found a correlation between serum levels in infants and the amount of "quiet" restorative sleep, comparing the effect to that achieved with barbiturates. Quiet sleep is non-REM sleep in which the baby is as still as a stone. That sounds fine to me.

Subsequent studies on men and women find ample evidence that magnesium deficiency leads to insomnia or sleep problems, and if you correct the deficiency, you correct the disorder. Sleep does come to magnesium-deficient people, of course (or most of us would never rest), but it may be more disorganized. There's evidence that low-mag people have less restorative REM sleep and more frequent waking, which researchers often chalk up to an overactive NMDA receptor (the one that magnesium usually guards), or another artifact of stress. If magnesium short-circuits the nervous response and prevents the NMDA receptor from becoming overexcited, the restless wee-hour mind has less fuel to run on. In one small Iranian study, men and women who took five hundred milligrams of magnesium daily for eight weeks also went to sleep more efficiently and had higher melatonin levels compared to a placebo group.

The most recent research suggests that magnesium helps cells cope with the natural environmental cycle of night and day. Every cell in the body has a "clock," and magnesium links the "clock genes" to the cycles of light and dark as well as the body's metabolism. Aligning the body to the solar day is an energy-saving tactic: cells can use more energy to produce more proteins during the day ("make hay while the sun shines") and then take a rest at night. In this way, magnesium may help set the clock that tells the body when it's time for sleep. When researchers at the University of Edinburgh removed magnesium from cells, it was as if the timepiece had sprung, and cells had longer circadian rhythms. It occurs to me that as daylight saving time kicks in and the days shift longer this time of year, the kids need to settle in to sleep even though it feels earlier. One more incentive to top up on magnesium: to set the body clock for the growing season.

This very evening, UJ goes to bed with a belly full of broccoli rabe and feet slightly sticky with magnesium salts. As she starts to drift off, I click off the light and peek around the window shade. Outside, a spring breeze blows through the trees. In the dim light of the streetlamp I can see that vines are starting to climb the brownstones on the other side of the street again. Hundreds of miles away, beyond the city's borders, are the farmlands where the season's food is just now pushing up through the soil. I look upward into the urban haze. Somewhere out there, above and beyond the pollution, is interstellar dust, a mix of silicon, oxygen, aluminum—and magnesium. Stardust, the stuff that grounds us.

MAY

Can Green Help
Gray Matter?

———

Kids are required to focus more than ever.
Can nature help mind wanderers?

THE ABILITY TO pay attention—to track what's going on, to stick
to a task—is invaluable. It's the other side of the coin—daydreaming—that is said to have dubious worth.

She's a daydreamer, UJ's teachers have always said. *Your kid spends*
too much time gazing out the window. Don't be mistaken. When she's
on, she's really on. She's deep. But when she's off, we're talking deep
space. We can't reach her. Earth to UJ!

So, I sit my daughter down one cloudless May morning. I hold
her soft hands in mine and look straight into her gray-green eyes.
"Wisdom," I say, "is knowing that there's a time for focus and a time

to dream. At school, it's time to focus." She gives a dismissive nod and looks down.

Several days later, at dinner, Peter has the same talk with her. "If you want to daydream in school, it's OK," he advises. "But it has to be volitional." She looks confused. "You have to do it by *choice*." She looks down at her plate.

She looks out the window, the teachers say.

"What do you see out the window?"

Construction. Tar. Brick. Rooftops. Pigeons. Beige, gray, black.

This is her view of the world.

Many young children fall into UJ's camp. They're not always on; they zone out, act out. UJ can concentrate so deeply on a puzzle that Ami's shrieks don't derail her. She can read a book from cover to cover in an evening. But then, especially in the middle of a school day, there's a siren song outside and she needs to attend to it.

Is this a good or a bad thing? My wish for her is to develop the ability to come back to Earth when necessary, and on her own. But maybe she must first go out there, far out there, to come back here.

The following is a chronicle of an outing.

Daydreaming is its own reward. For regardless of the result (if any), the very process of daydreaming is pleasurable. —Michael Pollan

Every Friday I pick up UJ from school. These walks home from school are meant to be bonding time, precious and painstakingly arranged. On this particular May afternoon, I'm holding her hand and asking her questions, thoughtful ones, about her day. "Any interesting math problems today? What are you studying in science—worms still? What was the silliest thing someone did in class? If you could change the day, what would you have done?" She begins, then trails off. She repeats phrases. She speaks in mosaics. She's brittle. She's vague.

Our worlds are drifting apart, hers and mine. Now that she's in kindergarten she spends most of her waking hours away from me. Her arms are folded against her chest as if she were in a straitjacket. She turns away from me and glances skyward. This after-school behavior is happening more and more frequently, and I'm distressed. She doesn't want to talk and she doesn't want me to talk. She's tapped out.

Time to experiment.

"How about we go to the park?" I say.

I'd like to know if a thirty-minute stint among the robins and London plane trees might make any difference at all in terms of restoring her attention when she's particularly dazed. By now, spring has truly sprung, the daffodils are blooming, and the park looks like something out of a fairy tale. "Let's go," I say, and she nods solemnly. I take her hand as we enter at the southwest corner, passing pretzel carts and a man operating a tiny drone.

Two minutes into the greenery, UJ finds a low railing and walks, arms out, tightrope-walker style. "How was your day? What did you do?" I ask again. Wobblingly, she speaks. "I read *Pandora's Box*. Ummm. I made a marble run. Ummm. Played chess. Umm. Painted a beach scene with, like, like . . . like a frame. In arts and crafts. And, and, and . . . and we played a pattern game called Sequence."

Some information is better than no information, but there's no flow. The signal is only coming through in blips and bleeps.

So I tune in to the metamessage.

Every activity she mentions, even perhaps the art, falls into the category of what the late nineteenth-century psychologist William James called directed attention. They all involve listening up, hunkering down, switching tasks and transitioning, leaning in, or shutting up when told. To do any of these tasks, a child must filter out distractions and maintain focus.

"Did you finish your work at school today?" I ask.

No answer. Her attention is directed everywhere else, which is to say it is not directed attention.

The early lilacs became part of this child, / And grass, and white and red morning-glories, and white and red clover, and the song of the phoebe-bird. —Walt Whitman

William James might have said that my five-year-old's attention is exactly where it should be. The mind of a young child (presumably the under-ten set), he said, is naturally in a state of imaginative and undirected attention. You can call it daydreaming or mind-wandering, in which one thought flows spontaneously to the next. In neuroscience circles, it's called the "default mode." Whatever you call it, it's mental downtime, but not the sort spent reading or building towers or singing, which all draw on directed attention even when done for pleasure. Even watching TV involves tuning in. The default mode is a different channel: the gaze falls into the mid-distance, seeing without focusing on anything specific. It's the last refuge of the young child who's no longer carefree.

There is something else that undirected attention, or the default mode, is not. It is the opposite of mindfulness, which we value so much these days. I'm always telling UJ to be mindful—of what's in her hands, of whether her chin is over her plate, of where her limbs are in relation to a cup or another person's body, and of what she needs to do next. *What's next, sweetie?* Mindfulness involves purposefulness and moment-by-moment awareness. But it's quite possibly overvalued in children.

When daydreaming, there's no *next*, no logical sequence. Memories, random bits of information, reflections, hypothetical situations, future scenarios, future selves, fantasies, anything—it all moves in an easy, haphazard flow from one to the next. James observed that this state "makes a child seem to belong less to himself than to every object which happens to catch his notice." There are no boundaries, no magnetic center. In this description, James seemed to be channeling my favorite Walt Whitman poem, "There Was a Child Went Forth": "And the first object he looked upon . . . , that object he became. / And that object became part of him for the day, or a certain part of the day, or for many years, or stretching cycles of years." It's a state of pure absorption.

Once in the park, UJ looked upon the crisp green grass stretched out before her, and that grass she became. She batted the stems of flowers, and those flowers she became. She swung on a low bough of a pine tree, and that tree she became. She twirled with her arms outstretched like her new idol, Maria in *The Sound of Music*, her purple velvet skirt with sequined ladybugs and bees flaring. She streamed her force field.

It occurs to me how achingly precious this downtime is for her. I think I speak for most American kids that are elementary-school age and older when I say that there's not much bandwidth for dreamy reverie anymore. We don't have the time, or make the time, between school's out and lights out. There's homework, music practice, sports practice, dinner, dishes, bath time, reading time. For older kids, there are also after-school activities, religious groups, clubs, and part-time jobs. There's no free time.

While the freeform, inward-looking default mode isn't mindfulness, it's not fair to say it's *mindlessness*. It may look like the lights are on but no one's home, but real-time fMRI scans of daydreamers reveal a lot going on in the basement, far below the level of our conscious awareness. A few brain regions are unexpectedly "on" and very active: the medial prefrontal cortex, which reacts to social and emotional information and tries to make sense of it; the hippocampus, which generates memories; the posterior cingulate cortex, which integrates memory retrieval; and the amygdala, which gives rise to emotions. Although there's some overlap between the default network and the focused-attention network, the other key areas of the brain involved in concentration are, as you might expect, turned off.

One way to look at default mode is as mental energy running helter-skelter, liberated from the normal constraints of directed attention. It's the circuitry of creativity. A switch fires and something ignites: spontaneous thoughts, ruminations, runaway emotions. It's an electric eureka in the morning shower. It's the effortless fountain of ideas. The mind is sifting and recombining bits of information, making unexpected connections between complex ideas, and meaning-making, as in REM dream sleep. Sometimes it is even running problem-solving simulations far under the radar of conscious awareness to prepare for landing back in reality.

The only real valuable thing is intuition. —Albert Einstein

Here's an exercise for your kid. Ask him or her to sit down at a table with a paper and pencil and come up with as many uses as possible for a brick. This classic creativity test is named, rather unimaginatively, the Unusual Uses Task. The goal is to come up with the most unique ideas. The kid has two minutes. Ready, set, go.

How many uses did your child (or you) think up? How innovative are they? Several years ago, a trio of researchers at the University of California at Santa Barbara—Benjamin Baird, Jonathan Smallwood, and Jonathan Schooler—used the Unusual Uses Task in an experiment. First they presented the brick challenge (and others) to their subjects, asking them to come up with their most creative ideas. Everyone scored about the same.

Then, between trials, the subjects were divided into four groups. The first group had to undertake memory and reaction-time tasks for twelve minutes, the second got to simply rest for the same amount of time, and a third group had no break. Meanwhile, the fourth group had a soul-crushingly boring twelve-minute assignment in which they had to watch a stream of black numbers pass by until they saw one that was colored and an even number, in which case they'd press a button. This activity was so tedious that everyone's mind wandered after a few minutes.

Citizen scientists, subject your child to a boring activity for twelve minutes. It need not be as dull as a number stream—just any task that requires little focus. Science has found several other surefire ways to induce mind-wandering: throw a rubber ball at the wall repeatedly, read a book that's too dense (*War and Peace* is popular in these studies), listen to a monotone lecture, wash dishes, look out the window, take a shower. When the twelve minutes are up, give the kid the same Unusual Uses challenge as the students in the study. *Try again to come up with unique uses for a brick.* How many can your child think up now?

In the UC Santa Barbara study, the group that was given a boring task and daydreamed for twelve minutes came up with 41 percent more original ideas for the brick in the second round than did the other groups. *It's soap! It's a catapult! A stage for bugs! A butt warmer!*

So, what was going on in those twelve minutes of boredom? If you asked the thinkers, they might have said they were zoning out. What they didn't realize is that part of their brain seemed to be still mulling over the challenge and generating new unconscious associations and wild ideas. When the thinkers came back online, the ideas surfaced to conscious awareness. Note, the combustive moment comes only from having a question or a problem in mind, going offline to incubate it, then going back online to think about it again. When the daydreamers were given a *new* challenge in the second round (*How many ideas can you come up with for a brown bag?*), they were no more creative than the other groups.

You might assume that your child will be more productive when he or she focuses on a problem, but that's not true for problems that are complex or require creativity. They need to use their powers of unfocused attention. One theory about the daydreamers' superior creativity is that in their spaced-out state their default networks were still mulling over new ways to repurpose a brick, and so were their "attention networks," which kept the goal in mind and brought it back to a conscious level. When these two usually opposing networks work in parallel, breakthroughs emerge. The brains of the most creative innovators show more activity in their default-mode network all the time (especially between the frontal and parietal regions). They have more difficulty suppressing the cross talk between default mode regions. Albert Einstein, incidentally, was a notorious daydreamer.

The neuroscientist Mary Helen Immordino-Yang, a professor at the University of Southern California, suggests that creativity is one of the two cherished qualities that come of daydreaming. The second we should hold equally dear: introspection. When people daydream, Immordino-Yang found, the same neural circuitry switches on as when people are asked to process or reflect on abstract social, moral, or emotional ideas.

Take, for instance, the dialogue between Immordino-Yang's team and a college-age volunteer during one of their experiments. The volunteer was told to reflect on a story he had just read about a starving single mother and her son. The son wants his mama to eat, but she lies, saying she has already had enough because she wants him to fill his own belly without guilt. When the researchers asked their subject how he felt about the story, he started out by summarizing it. Then he paused—and that pause, suggests Immordino-Yang, was the default network kicking in for a moment. A flash of insight, and the next thing they knew he was on a very different track. *I don't thank my own family enough.*

Immordino-Yang found that the more a person pauses when talking about prosocial emotions—a signal of a momentary switch to the default network—the more complex and cognitively abstract his or her thinking. We all revere deep thinking, but we need to make space for it. Just as American culture so often values extroverted behavior over introverted, so we value "looking out" more than "looking in." If kids are told that they always need to stay focused on the external world, that they shouldn't pause for reflection, or if they're always entertained by video games, texts, and TV, then they don't dip so much into the default mode. They miss out on that deeper introspective thinking. Do they fail to develop the skills to think creatively and reflectively? That's the worry.

Focused attention will get a child to think about "what happened" or "how to do this," Immordino-Yang writes in her study, "Rest Is Not Idleness." But unfocused attention, she explains, lends itself to "what this means for the world and for the way I live my life." Only deeper, more emotionally engaged thinking leads to meaning making. To paraphrase Immordino-Yang, a kid isn't going to care about something she hasn't thought deeply about, and she isn't going to think deeply about something she doesn't care about.

A daydreamer is prepared for most things. —Joyce Carol Oates

Not all mind-wandering gets you to a summit. Sometimes you end up in the pits, found Harvard psychologists Daniel Gilbert and Matthew Killingsworth, whose research linked it with the onset of negative moods. Sometimes you get stuck in a negative loop. The urge to let your mind wander may come from boredom, stress, or unhappiness. It may be a sign of burned-out working memory, which is the ability to stay focused while juggling tasks. Some daydreams are clearly better than others, and the difference might have everything to do with mood and context.

Can we use nature to deepen the default mode and thus maximize the prized bounce back in attention? I have a suspicion that daydreaming while sitting in the classroom may not be as restorative as daydreaming while walking on the street. (The heart pumps faster, bringing blood and oxygen to organs, including the brain.) And daydreaming while walking on the street may not be as restorative as daydreaming while observing the motion of leaves blowing in the wind, shifting clouds, ripples, shadows, patterns in the grass, an explosion of flowers, the texture of a springtime meadow.

For further insight, I turn to a well-known Scottish study that used a portable device called an electroencephalogram to measure brain waves. The gadget can reveal when the mind is in an active or a restorative mode. In the study, subjects strolled through leafy green plazas and parks, much like the bushy-but-busy city park stroll I'm on with UJ, and their thoughts became expansive, attentive, and meditative. Twenty-five minutes later—or about a half mile into the stroll—the walkers said they felt restored and refreshed, and their brain-wave patterns backed them up. They looked like gentle undulations—tsunamis no more. The brains of urban walkers showed no such cognitive renewal.

To further test nature's efficacy in restoring attention, researchers at the University of Michigan tried to pulverize their volunteers' focus and concentration by asking them to count numbers backward, suppress their short-term memory for long periods of time, and other tasks (surely nothing more demanding than a day in a modern kindergarten). Then two groups were randomly assigned to take a nearly hour-long stroll through either a tree-lined park or downtown Ann Arbor past university and office buildings.

The researchers didn't quantify daydream time, but after the walk, the groups were asked to perform further tasks that required directed attention, like mental math. The walk refreshed both groups, but the nature strollers enjoyed a 19 percent improvement on memory and attention tests, compared to only a 6 percent boost among those who went for an urban stroll. Unlike in natural settings, the authors say, "urban environments require directed attention, making them less restorative."

Nature walks also reduce elevated blood glucose more than urban walks do, a Japanese study found. Better glucose regulation improves performance on cognitive and self-regulatory tasks. (Bear this in mind for the kid who drinks too much juice and eats too many crackers and other simple carbs.) While any exercise lowers blood sugar levels, a nature immersion soothes the vagus nerve, slows down blood pressure and heart rate, and, pointedly, lowers the hormone cortisol, which otherwise increases sugar in the blood. Credit the immersiveness of the experience, the sights and textures of plants and trees, even the phytoncides and microbes in the air. Maybe it's the *M. vaccae*. Nothing you can pinpoint precisely.

But if greenery is a biohack, even a microdose might do in a pinch. I was surprised to learn that students perform better on attention tests and stress recovery simply by being in a classroom with a green view. To be clear, just a view of greenery outside led to better focus than did the same setting with a view of built spaces (like UJ's urban classroom). Even if the greenery doesn't put students in default mode for long or at all, it acts like visual Valium.

If we were to peer into the brain, explains Colin Ellard at the University of Waterloo's Urban Realities Lab, we'd see that opioid ("reward") receptors in the brain's parahippocampal region respond with gusto to the sight of greenery. This area is important because it's part of the emotional (limbic) system, and it plays a role in memory formation. What makes nature so restorative and mesmerizing, the theory goes, is that it's fractal. Trees are natural fractals. Look at them closely and you'll see that they repeat smaller and smaller patterns of themselves. Buds made of smaller and smaller buds do too, as well as pinecone seeds and fern fronds and ice crystals. They all repeat themselves. These patterns hold our attention effortlessly and may shepherd us more easily into a restorative default mode. We blink less often when looking at them, which, Ellard says, is a sign of lower cognitive load and stress.

There are dozens of studies like these, all supporting the notion that nature, compared to other settings, offers a superior dip into default mode, which helps to restore attention and make creativity possible. Outdoor sights and sounds are subconscious triggers—the green bloom of flora, the woods dripping after rain, a field of dandelions, a gentle breeze, a firefly-lit evening. Daydreaming is a retreat into the increasingly endangered forest of one's own mind.

The cost of oblivious daydreaming was always this moment of return, the realignment with what had been before and now seemed a little worse. —Ian McEwan

At the half-hour mark at the park, my kid is, if anywhere, lost afield. I check in, and she still doesn't want to talk about her day or anything else. But before I let her slip away again into the gold and green, I take her hand in mine and tell her about the research on daydreaming. I do all the talking. The mind-wandering has become an issue lately, I say, but I tell her that it's OK. I repeat my mantra about the importance of time and place, and that there are times to focus and times to get blurry, like right after school. I ask her to try to catch herself in a daydream: awareness is the first step in managing them and harnessing them for creativity. "And if you have a good idea, capture it! Try to remember it for later." The underlying message is that daydreaming is OK, even good. As she listens, she visibly relaxes. I am saying something relieving.

Finally, she takes in a deep breath and responds. Now that the daydreaming license has been granted, I think she might be ready to talk about her day. Or maybe the scientific research.

"There's a tiny little tree, Mama, at school," she says, then trails off. She frowns.

"A tiny little tree . . . ?"

"Yes. And when I was there I was thinking a bird died and is buried under it."

I hold her hand tighter. "What do you mean, sweetie?"

At recess, she says, at the perimeter of the blacktop, there's a little bush that has just started to sprout green leaves. She likes to dig at the roots with a stick. That's what she does in her free time. With a shiver, I wonder if the bush is her shrine.

Biohack: Improving the School Daze

So powerful is nature's ability to restore attention that even tiny, homeopathic doses might help children focus a little longer. If a whiff of nature and a microescape helps mood, creativity, and attention, schools should consider these easy fixes:

- *Allow time and place for a real mind-wander.* My daughter now has "mindfulness" time at school, her absolute favorite activity, which she uses to do the opposite: mind-wander. No matter. Schools should find time and a place to allow or even encourage daydreaming. Prime daydreaming conditions can be created at home by making electronic gadgets, games, and possibly even books off-limits for a spell. Bonus for a window seat or sill on which to sit and gaze out at greenery.
- *Greenify the view.* The mere sight of greenery has a visceral effect on us. In one study, girls who lived in a public housing development in Chicago's South Side and had a room with a view of trees, bushes, or water—again, *just a view*—scored higher in concentration abilities and in impulse inhibition compared to their peers who looked out at blacktop and urban sprawl from their apartment windows. The suggestion of nature reduces sympathetic nervous activity (fight-or-flight response) and increases parasympathetic (rest-and-digest) activity, which promotes better health and self-control. In the classroom, it's not hard to put plants in the window, on the inside sill, or in window boxes outside.

- *Crack the window or door.* Every body in the room exhales carbon dioxide—and as CO_2 levels rise, so does inattention. This isn't healthy mind-wandering—it's more like straight-up oxygen deprivation. The result: mistakes, slips, foul tempers, and brain farts. The average classroom has CO_2 levels at around 1,000 ppm (outdoor levels are about 350 ppm), which isn't a killer, but a study at the University of California at Berkeley found that when students breathe for two hours at those "normal" levels, they make worse decisions than when in a room with lower CO_2 levels. By 2,500 ppm—a stuffier room in which kids might smell their classmates—brainpower was sapped. Specifically, participants' scores for "taking initiative," "thinking strategically," and "utilizing information" plummeted as carbon dioxide concentration increased, and attention was only restored after the windows were cracked and the doors opened. (Imagine how unfair it would be to take a standardized test in this setting.) The EPA guidelines for classrooms are set for CO_2 levels to be no higher than 1,000 ppm, but the recent studies suggest that by the time everyone is deeply breathing this air, their minds are long gone. Children need a breath of fresh air, literally and figuratively. Note: CO_2 meters cost about $100.
- *Take an after-school "green" break.* Aim for a twenty-minute walk through any green space. Let the kid's mind go free-range (and the body too, if possible). The goal is restored attention and creativity. At a minimum, the green walk should decrease cortisol levels, sympathetic nervous system activity, and blood pressure and increase heart rate variability (see chapter 12).

For fun, try the Unusual Uses Task in nature versus an indoor setting. Is your child more creative post–nature immersion? Do you see a shift in his or her ability to focus? If your child is working on a creative assignment, consider a green mind-wandering break first.

What scene better captures the essence of childhood than a child blowing the downy head off a dandelion? Legend has it that the number of breaths it takes to blow off all the fluff is the hour of the day. UJ blows on dandelions so hard that it's never later than three o'clock.

Despite all the pro-daydreaming evidence on my mind, I can't resist the knee-jerk impulse to engage one last time. "What's the dandelion's strategy?" I hear myself asking. As a science educator, I want UJ to think about why the dandelion looks the way it does. Can she figure out why the plant evolved to look like this? I need her to understand how the tiny seeds will disseminate when the fluff catches the wind, like little parachutes, and take root somewhere far away.

No response. UJ abruptly picks another dandelion and blows hard.

The moment seems ripe for the Unusual Uses Task, but this time with our own little twist.

"Hey," I say in a gently challenging voice. "What all the uses you can come up with for dandelion fluff? You have two minutes. Be super creative."

That pulls her out of her reverie. "Um. Mattress stuffing," she says.

"More."

"Pillow stuffing."

"Doesn't count." I sigh. "Needs to be unique."

"Fake snow . . . bird feathers . . ."

She trails off, picking at the seeds on her shirt, rolling them around in her fingers absently. I've lost her again.

"Time's up!" I chirp. That didn't go as well as I'd hoped.

My daughter begins talking to herself with mounting enthusiasm. "The softest of fluff!" she shouts, citing Dr. Seuss's *Sleep Book* in which a creature called the Jed grows pom-poms for his bed. She throws the dandelion seeds into the air. "Wheee!" She collects fluff, puts it in her pockets, and turns her head this way and that, on the lookout for new specimens. She's chattering about the Cupids, her imaginary legion of magical beings. They'll save our polluted planet's animals and can spin dandelion fluff into silk kimonos.

I look at my phone. We've been outside for forty-seven minutes. "Time to go, sweetie."

No response.

I'm dimly aware that UJ is slipping in and out of a streaming default mode while I'm still stuck in directed attention, looking for ways to optimize and maximize her childhood. What does she know that I don't? This: one should not bring a kid to nature with the expectation that her attention will be restored immediately, or even quickly. There's no magical twenty-five-minute threshold, despite what the studies suggest. A kid must get away for an indefinite amount of time before she can come back. You can't put a timer on it.

So I spend seven more minutes watching my child honor every dandelion seed. She touches them. Rolls them, rolls in them. Gets them under her fingernails. There's an easy flow to the moment. The softest of fluff, moving in the direction of a gentle wind, falling wherever it may.

It'll take root when it's ready.

And so, on the way home, I ask the dandelion fluff question one more time. "How many weird uses can you think of for the stuff?" She's holding my hand, swinging it, and now the ideas come forth: "Glue, fake snow, Father Time beard, starry universe, time travel, fake insects, goose down substitute, magical potion . . ."

JUNE

Eternal Springtime of the Flavonoid Mind

Are blues the tastiest of memory hacks?

MY DAUGHTER SITS at the table, batting the air dismissively. Before her is a white shatterproof bowl. The kid knows that the fruit is part of our new experiment with flavonoids, which are powerful plant chemicals. She knows that she's supposed to eat them. The problem is, a cup and half of blueberries is a lot to eat in a sitting.

I do what any other parent might do under duress: I bribe. "Eat," I say, "and later you'll get something you like. *Chocolate.*"

Flavonoids are the plant dyes that make blueberries deep blue, oranges orange, cocoa beans brown. If you're a berry growing in a high altitude, your deep violet-blue tint protects you from the sun's ultraviolet light. If you're fruit or vegetable or flower, having a deep or bright color saves your skin and attracts pollinators. Flavonoids protect plants from other stresses too—extreme heat and cold, salty and acidic soils, and heavy metals—in part by altering the soil composition, which in turn influences the plant's metabolism or immunity. Broadly speaking, the more adverse the plant's conditions, the deeper or more colorful it is and the more flavonoids it produces. Blue is arguably the most potent hue of all.

I tell UJ that she's lucky to freeload on the fruits of botanical resilience. When we eat high-flavonoid foods our circulation is better, our immune system stronger, our neurons more resistant to inflammation. Vitamins are better transported through our bloodstream, our detoxification pathways are stronger, and our cell cycle balance is better regulated so that mutations are fewer and when one cell dies, another replaces it. Just as flavonoids protect the plant's skin from the sun, they protect ours too, visibly slowing down the aging of the epidermis (not that my kid cares about this yet, but I do). And none of this yet touches on the potential brain benefits that inspire the blueberry experiment we're about to do.

Of the more than four thousand flavonoids identified so far, the predominant ones in blueberries belong to a class called anthocyanins, which are singled out for their fabled memory-boosting abilities. Any bluish-reddish-purplish fruit or vegetable you can think of—blackberries, bilberries, red cabbages, black currants, cherries, eggplants, red onions—contain anthocyanins, but blueberries have among the highest levels. The wild ones in UJ's bowl grew in high elevations in acidic, sandy soil under the full Northern California sun—the right amount of stress for a tip-top anthocyanin concentration.

In lab experiments, befuddled old rats that were fed anthocyanins for several weeks suddenly navigated mazes and easily memorized the tricky locations where food was hidden. Senior citizens (humans) who'd complained of brain fog not only said they felt clearer after four months on a blueberry diet but also scored nearly 75 percent better when asked questions that drew on semantic memory, like *Who was president in 2000? What's the capital of Florida?* Multiple studies find the same trend: the more flavonoids people have in their diets, the sharper they are in old age.

My investigation, however, concerns memory and *young* brains. If blueberry juice can rejuvenate older brains, what effect might it have on young, developing brains?

It would be easy to jack up kids on anthocyanin extract powders or pills, then test their memory. Problem is, at least in people, flavonoids don't seem to perform their magic in isolation. Anthocyanins in particular work best when they interact with other plant chemicals that enhance our ability to absorb or process them but that aren't themselves bioactive. This is a *whole food* story.

Sorry, UJ. You've got to eat that whole darn bowl of berries.

You don't remember what happened. What you remember becomes what happened. —John Green

Imagine that your kid, like mine, just ate a cup and a half of blueberries. Now the bowl is gone, and you're sitting across from him or her and holding a sheet of paper with several lists of words. Each list has fifteen words, and you ask your child to listen to each of them, all unrelated nouns, at the rate of one word per second. Immediately after you're finished, he or she must think back and tell you all the words he or she can remember, in any order. This gold-standard test is called RAVLT, short for Rey Auditory Verbal Learning Test, and it measures short-term memory.

Ready? Read the following words carefully. (Or, to test yourself, just read the words below, one by one, then cover them up.)

A List

shirt	apple	carton	dog	drum	school	garden	moon
farmer	nose	river	color	curtain	hat	turkey	

How many words did your child remember? Read the list again
(or read it again yourself, then cover it up). How many can he or
she remember now? Subjects should do a little better each time
they hear the list, naturally. Your kid gets five recall rounds, which
means he or she gets to hear the list five times. By the fifth round
your guinea pig might remember two or three more words than in
the first round.

But don't get too confident. There's a twist. Before the sixth round
your kid gets to hear another list of words, which is also read out loud,
one per second. This is called the B list, and it's meant to muddy one's
memory. It's an interference list.

B List

bread	door	lemon	card	desk	glasses	towel	lamb
gun	fish	school	mountain	shoes	bird	hair	

Now see if you child can remember these new words. Not so
good, right? Most people have a harder time remembering words in
the B list than in the first round of the A list. Speaking of which, it's
time to see how many words from the A list your subject can still
remember. It's OK to either say them or write them down. This is
the sixth time your kid is trying to remember these words, and he or
she doesn't get to hear them again this time.

"How many did you remember?" you'll ask. "Did you remember
eight words? Ten? Did you do as well as you did before you heard the
B list?" Probably not. There's usually a big dip here in the number of

words recalled because it's hard to remember the A list after hearing the B list.

Wait fifteen minutes and ask your subject to try again. This is the delayed recall round. How many A-list nouns do you remember now? Even fewer, right? (If you'd like to challenge your child to take your version of the RAVLT, see the text box on page 117 for further details).

The RAVLT is one test in a battery of cognitive assessments that Claire Williams, a neuroscientist at the University of Reading in England, gave to a group of schoolkids. Officially, the RAVLT measures explicit declarative memory, which is to say it measures how well we remember something immediately after we learn it, in the near future, and even in the presence of distracting, irrelevant information.

Williams and her colleagues, Adrian Whyte and Graham Schafer, applied a variation of the RAVLT to see if the anthocyanins and other flavonoids in blueberries might help strengthen memory in seven- to twelve-year-olds, an age group when children experience a spurt in frontal lobe growth. Not many researchers study children, Williams says, because kids already function at a high level and an improvement in performance might not show up on most tests. If Williams could show that children also perform better on cognitive tests after eating blueberries, her research would be among the first to prove the potency (and potential) of these plant chemicals on the developing brain.

This would be an important finding. Better short-term memory might help children remember a paragraph they just read or a new vocabulary word or a step in a mathematical equation. They'd have a better chance of being able to make real-time links between new and old information. There's an undeniable connection between short-term memory and the ability to learn and make meaning.

Williams and her group at the University of Reading's nutritional psychology lab staged an experiment in a school cafeteria. They divided the twenty-one kids into three groups and gave each group one of three drinks: a shake with thirty grams of wild blueberry powder (the equivalent to 240 grams, or 1½ cups, of fresh wild blueberries containing 253 milligrams of anthocyanins); a fifteen-gram wild blueberry powder drink (equivalent to 120 grams or ¾ cup fresh wild blueberries with 127 milligrams of anthocyanins plus extra sugar and vitamin C to match the thirty-gram drink); or a low-flavonoid drink with the same amount of sugar and vitamin C to match the other two drinks. Each day for three days, Williams asked the children to gulp down their assigned drinks and take the RAVLT and other tests. She'd test them at baseline, and then again at one hour and fifteen minutes; then at three hours; then again at six hours after consuming their assigned drinks.

What Williams hoped to glean is whether the blueberries would somehow boost kids' performance on the RAVLT and other memory tests. If so, how soon until you see an effect? She knew from the tests on mice and human adults that a powerful dose of anthocyanins might make some difference in learning. Then again, a child's brain is a somewhat different animal.

Memory is the mother of all wisdom. —Aeschylus

An hour and fifteen minutes after eating the cup and a half of blueberries, UJ listens to the fifteen words I made up as an A list. She presses her fingers into her eye sockets. She wrinkles her brow. "Card, lemon, farm, orchid, lamp . . ." By the fifth time she hears the words she remembers ten of the fifteen words, which is the same as her baseline before she ate blueberries. She remembers nine A-list words after hearing the B list. She remembers ten words from the A list after the fifteen-minute delay. Not bad. For delayed recall, she does about as well or slightly better than her baseline test this morning right before eating blueberries. She remembers about one word more in each round than when she did in a previous control experiment with an orange drink that had zero anthocyanins in it. (To try to avoid bias, I told her that the drink was as good for her memory as blueberries.)

When I test UJ's memory with a new A and B list three hours after baseline, she remembers fewer words overall than at the hour-and-fifteen-minute mark, which can happen, but I think it bothers her. So, at the six-hour test I note that she's looking at me with an expression of real interest. Her fingers are on her temples. I read the list—"Wheel, fan, teeth, horse . . ."—and a grin spreads on her face. Suddenly it seems the RAVLT is fun, and in this round she has her best performance by far, even exceeding her morning baseline. She remembers twelve of the fifteen words by the fifth time she hears the list, and nine words after the distracting B list interference. What stands out for UJ at this six-hour mark is her performance on the fifteen-minute delayed recall. She remembers twelve A-list words. That's four words more than she remembered in this section than on the day without blueberries, which is pretty striking.

Let's look at how the kids in Williams's study did on their RAVLTs. Their baseline tests were at 8:30 in the morning before they had the blueberry (or control) drink. Like UJ, most kids remembered about nine or ten words by the fifth time they heard the A list, and everyone remembered fewer words (about eight) right after listening to and having to recall the words on the B list, and about the same after a fifteen-minute delay. As you might expect, the kids' performance on these tests declined over the day. Fatigue creeps in and a ghost memory of words from earlier lists interferes with the recollection of new lists.

Now here's the interesting part. By the one-hour-fifteen-minute mark, the blueberry kids consistently remembered about one more word each round than the control group did. The group that had the megadose (one and a half cups), like my daughter, scored the best overall. The advantage showed up in each testing period—at an hour fifteen, three hours, and six hours (although the group was stronger at an hour fifteen and six hours for delayed recall). In the test that the kids took six hours after the baseline, those who ate either the small or large portion of berries remembered almost two words more on average than kids in the control group—that's a lot on this test. In the delayed recall round, the blueberry eaters recalled at least a word more (about six) than the tapped-out control group.

The blueberry eaters' memories were a little stickier.

Out of fifteen words on a list, a few more caught and held in memory's net doesn't sound so astounding, but from a scientific perspective it's meaningful. It suggests that something about blueberries helps us to encode memory, and this advantage might show up in real-life learning. The schoolchildren not only were able to acquire and recognize words a bit better after eating blueberries but also did a generally better job in overcoming the interference of new information (the B list). Williams notes that the high-dose blueberry group also did better on some of her other tests, including a selective attention test that required kids to ignore distractors. (However, blueberries appeared to do nothing for spatial memory or response inhibition in this study, unlike similar ones on adults.)

For Williams, the outcome of this experiment was validating. It backed up a smaller trial she had previously published. In that study, eight- to ten-year-olds ate a two-hundred-gram dose of blueberries, and just two hours later, they were better at retaining words after a twenty-five-minute delay than non–blueberry eaters. The blueberries in that study were the farmed variety you'd find at the grocery store year-round.

We are that strange species that constructs artifacts intended to counter the natural flow of forgetting. —William Gibson

If I had the tools to peer into my blueberry eater's brain, I'd see a lot more blood flowing up there than usual. The Nobel Prize winner who discovered flavonoids in the 1930s, Albert Szent-Györgyi, was initially struck by the ability of flavonoids to dilate and strengthen capillaries and improve vascular function—that is, circulation. The big idea now is that anthocyanins and flavanols (another class of flavonoid) can cross the blood-brain barrier to increase blood flow within the cerebral arteries in the brain. This includes the prefrontal cortex, which is associated with emotional regulation and cognitive control. It also includes those areas in the hippocampus where memory is stored. A stronger blood flow carries in more oxygen and nutrients, which in turn strengthen the synapses, the junctures between neurons where information is passed and stored.

What does this have to do with memory? Well-nourished synapses are plastic, meaning that they're able to reshape themselves in response to new knowledge. The more synaptic plasticity, the more a person can memorize and learn. To paraphrase Heraclitus, "You can't step in the same river twice, for it's not the same river and you're not the same person," and so it goes with the learning brain. It isn't the same brain from day to day, as synapses are ever changing, strengthening and weakening with experience. When there are more anthocyanins in the diet, there's also more brain blood flow, and then more brain-derived neurotrophic factor (BDNF), informally known as "Miracle-Gro." BDNF makes synaptic plasticity possible, which in turn strengthens the memory. Previous research found that peak cerebral blood flow occurs between one to two hours after a dose of flavonoids. That happens to be around the time when blueberry-dosed kids start to outperform their non-blueberry-eating peers in word recall tests.

By itself, increased blood flow to the brain may be sufficient explanation for the blueberry boost we see in children. But Williams and other researchers think there's another way that flavonoids, and anthocyanins in particular, strengthen the ability to learn and concentrate. The anthocyanins themselves, or the chemicals they're broken down into, may pass through the blood-brain barrier. Rat experiments show that anthocyanins are detectable in the brain in as few as ten minutes after consumption. There, they can directly stimulate the production of BDNF or stabilize BDNF levels in the hippocampus. The process of encoding, storing, and recalling the trace of a memory depends on BDNF. Without it, memories are unstable and fuzzy. Not much of what we experience would stick.

Memories are formed in the hippocampus, and a kid's budding hippocampus is especially sensitive to diet and environment. It'd be good for my daughters' hippocampi to have a lot of BDNF, I think, and I wonder if there's any hard evidence that anthocyanins can boost levels. You can't look at the hippocampus tissue of your kid, but studies on martyred young rats that have been fed anthocyanins show that yes, they have significantly higher levels of BDNF and springlike signs of neurogenesis in the memory region than their untreated peers. Naturally, the rats with the higher BDNF levels also had better spatial and long-term memories in their short lives.

Switching over to humans, a study on young adults found that BDNF levels in blood plasma (which reflect BDNF in brain tissue) rise as quickly as one hour after consuming the equivalent of two hundred grams of fresh blueberries. Improved memory effects emerged at two different time points: around one and a half hours and five hours, but not at the three-hour mark, which says something about how anthocyanins in blueberries are digested, absorbed, and metabolized. (Note that my daughter recalled fewer words at the three-hour mark than at other time points.)

Guess what determines how well each of us metabolizes anthocyanins? Are you thinking microbes? Incidentally, the anthocyanins and dietary fiber in blueberries are favorite foods of *Bifidobacterium*, which flourish in a blueberry gut. In one study, researchers formed two groups: every day, one group drank a wild blueberry drink consisting of twenty-five grams of powder (375 milligrams of anthocyanins) mixed with water, while the other group drank a non-blueberry drink. Six weeks later, bifidobacteria counts doubled in the blueberry group, while the untreated group's numbers stayed the same. *Doubled*, in part because anthocyanins create a low-oxidation environment favorable for microbes that are uniquely able to metabolize the plant compounds.

For each of us, our personal gut microbes may determine the extent to which blueberries—or any other food—nourish and boost us. And the blueberries, in turn, may determine how much of a Bifs boost we get. I begin to see the two as a supersynergic wit-grit duo: the anthocyanins give rise to better memory and learning, and *Bifidobacterium* contribute to stress resilience, spatial learning, memory, and more. Both trigger the BDNF surge we're all seeking.

Biohack: The Anthocyanin Challenge

The challenge is to get up to 200 milligrams of anthocyanins (about a cup of blueberries) in your kid, every day, or at least every few days. Bear in mind that the average person in the United States eats as little as 12.5 milligrams of anthocyanins a day. Making up the difference is a tall order.

The first hurdle is to determine the approximate anthocyanin load in the food you're serving. The anthocyanin concentration varies dramatically depending on the variety of fruit (wild blueberries have more than farmed ones, Williams says, because flavonoids are mostly in the skin of the fruits, and wild blueberries have a higher skin-to-flesh ratio) and the season and conditions under which the food was grown and stored. To my surprise there's evidence that frozen blueberries have more bioavailable anthocyanins than fresh berries because the ice crystals that form during the freezing process destroy the plant cell walls, thereby increasing the bioavailability of the contents. (This is good news for the wallet, too; frozen blueberries can be bought in bulk year-round and are dramatically cheaper than fresh ones.) For similar reasons, a study found that blanching—plunging the berries in boiling water for twenty-five to thirty seconds then removing them with a slotted spoon—also increases bioavailabilty. The blood plasma of blanched-blueberry eaters revealed even higher levels of anthocyanins than those who ate the berries fresh.

Fresh blueberries have a higher concentration of anthocyanins than dried or powdered blueberries. Powered extract, meanwhile, appears to yield more anthocyanin than juice. My daughters won't eat eggs without smothering them in blueberry jelly, but unfortunately the process of heating berries (in jams, jellies, juices, and purees) results in major flavonoid loss. The same goes for canning. The less processed, the better.

Because microbes help our bodies to absorb and break down anthocyanins, consider combining anthocyanin-rich foods with probiotic foods. Blueberry yogurt smoothies? Black raspberry kefir? Chokeberry kimchi?

How close can your kid get to 200 milligrams? Here's the approximate concentration of anthocyanins (in milligrams per 100 grams) in common food:

aubergine (eggplant)	750	cranberry	60–200
black currant	130–400	elderberry	450
blackberry	83–326	raspberry	365
blueberry	25–497	black raspberry	558
wild blueberry	558	red currant	80–420
cherry	350–400	red grape	30–750
chokeberry	200–1,000		

If you're curious to see if the blueberry memory boost works, try giving your kid your version of the RAVLT test as described earlier. To try to replicate Williams's experiment:

1. Think up four pairs of A and B lists, each with fifteen generic nouns.
2. Your subject gets to hear the words on the A list five times, and tries to recall as many words as possible each time. You keep track of the count.
3. Next, introduce the words on the B list and ask the child to remember as many of those words as possible.
4. Then ask you child to remember as many words as possible from the A list again. For the final, delayed recall round, wait fifteen minutes, then ask again.
5. Test your child four times during the day: right before eating either 1½ cups or ¾ cup of wild blueberries (whole or blended in a shake), then again at one hour and fifteen minutes, three hours, and six hours after consuming or drinking the blueberries. To be a little more scientific in your experimentation, establish a control by giving your kid a similarly sweet but anthocyanin-free drink on another day and try doing rounds of the memory recall at the same prescribed times as in the blueberry condition.

Did he or she do better at the hour-and-fifteen-minute and six-hour marks? How did memory compare on a blueberry-eating day versus a day without any flavonoids? How about after regular consumption for a few weeks? When my daughter took the RAVLT after eating blueberries about three to four times a week for four weeks (and on the test day), her score was even slightly higher on the delayed sections of the RAVLT than on the first blueberry-eating day, and consistently better than on the day earlier in the month when she tested without blueberries.

Remember, timing may be key to this biohack. If your child has a test or performance, have him or her eat at least ¾ cup blueberries (or other anthocyanin-rich foods) at least an hour beforehand. Peak levels of flavonoids are detected in the blood one to two hours and six hours following blueberry eating, which also corresponds to the times when their effects on cognitive tests are strongest. (With chocolate flavonoids, there is only one peak, two hours after consumption.) Plan accordingly.

Herewith is our dream program. Each morning kicks off with at least three-quarters of a cup of frozen wild blueberries. We're counting on a long-term payoff: a big memory cache. Maybe, just maybe, if a kid eats anthocyanins daily (the amount of the large dose in Williams's study) she'd grow a more BDNF-saturated synaptically plastic hippocampus than she would otherwise. Memory, after all, is the foundation of learning. My daughters would learn Spanish—or any other language—faster, because foreign words would stick better. They'd remember instructions. They'd recall directions forward and backward, dance steps, and do mental math at warp speed. They'd draw on facts and keep them straight even when barraged with new or distracting information.

It's worth mentioning that Ami, our youngest family member, has had at least a yearlong head start in this endeavor. She ravishes blueberries and other anthocyanin-rich fruit (blackberries, red grapes) with bank-breaking gusto. We call her the blueberry monster. Apocryphal as this is, Ami is as stress-resistant as any wild blueberry, and her memory is deep as the roots of ironweed. She remembers the location of my cell phone, her sister's sneakers, the keys. Something's missing? Ask the toddler, who'll deliver it with a fetching grin. At eighteen months old she'll recite colors and count to fifteen. "Just another artifact of an uncluttered mind," Peter says dismissively.

I can't prove it's the blueberries—yet. While the long-term effects of flavonoids on adult brains are well established, their role in shaping the structure of the hippocampus remains speculative. In childhood, the hippocampus is at a sensitive developmental stage, so it's possible that it stands to gain more from anthocyanins and the potential BDNF boosts they bring. (Meanwhile, young and middle-aged adults may gain more in frontal areas related to executive function.) It's not much of a stretch to see how increased blood flow to these areas of the brain during critical phases of development would help strengthen neural circuitry over the long term. However, to elevate blood flow and BDNF levels consistently enough to alter the structure and function of the hippocampus, a kid might need to eat blueberries every day for weeks or months. Could we possibly keep this up throughout childhood for the sake of a stronger memory? (Some studies report the hippocampus reaches peak volume at nine to eleven years old, although new neurons can grow there throughout life.) Theoretically, Williams says, positive changes in childhood could have a significant impact throughout life.

Williams's future research is practical. She wants to look at whether kids whose diets are supplemented with blueberries every day for several weeks or longer will show better cognitive function than kids who ate just one big short-term dose. If they do, it would support the idea that the accumulative effects of anthocyanins can shape early developmental pathways. Williams also wants to know how long the magic lasts and what happens when kids stop eating anthocyanins. "Will those positive changes in cognition persist for a few days, a few weeks, or longer term?"

I think you remember everything . . . you just can't bring it to mind all the time. —Edward Albee

Anthocyanins aren't the only memory-boosting flavonoids. Flavanols, the flavor of flavonoid in dark chocolate, are promising too. In a study conducted in Mexico City, where the pollution is as thick as black bean soup, inner-city children ate thirty grams of chocolate (a medium-sized bar) a day for about ten days. They performed better in short-term memory tests than the kids not fed chocolate, which the researchers attribute to flavanols that protect the neurons in the hippocampus from toxins.

To UJ's disappointment, children are hardly ever recruited in chocolate research. Grown men and women are subjects, and from these studies we have a bunch of findings to savor: People who eat about ten grams of chocolate daily for several weeks are sharper on memory tests. They're less likely to have dementia. They speak faster and more fluidly, have a better spatial working memory, and show a slowdown in the aging of the brain. (Good news for those afflicted with "Mommy Brain.") And yet, research on high-dose flavanols in cocoa find that the gain in attention and working memory may come at a cost: inaccuracy, which is often attributed to mental fatigue. There's a point at which the chocolate lover is perhaps too buzzed and sloppy, as chocolate also contains other compounds, such as caffeine and the stimulant theobromine. If there's any consensus in the chocolate research it's that long-term chocolate consumption (that is, eating it daily for a month) leads to *a better mood.*

On this measure, it's not fair to compare blueberries with chocolate, although research by Williams and others found that positive mood increases in children (in studies of seven- to ten-year-olds and young adults) two hours after consuming blueberries, regardless of time of day, whereas a placebo drink had no effect.

But eight hours after blueberries, my daughter is not in a better mood. She's grimly focused on making CrayCraks, a made-up currency that she says can only be used to buy pottery, and she doesn't particularly want to interact or be interrupted. Still, I ask her to take the memory test one extra time. Williams did not subject her subjects to an eight-hour test—the school day ended and kids went home—but I am curious to know if anthocyanins might have a long-lingering effect. UJ did so well at the six-hour mark. Had she been a bit more silver-tongued, even brighter and faster, or was it my imagination?

With weary resolve she agrees to take a final memory test of the day. It's six o'clock now, in early summer, and a shaft of liquid light pours on the sheet of paper before me. Last time. "Shirt, star, rugs, keys . . ."

She recalls up to eleven of the fifteen words over the next few rounds. After list B, she remembers ten words. After the fifteen-minute delay, she still remembers ten. Fantastic! At the same time of day on a non-blueberry day, she remembered only nine words after list B and eight words after the delay, which was about average. That's *eight hours* after eating the bowl of blueberries. She beams as if something great and transfiguring has occurred.

Like I've said before, our home experiments are anecdotes, not antidotes. There may be other reasons why UJ achieved similar results to the kids in Williams's lab-controlled studies and surpassed them in some rounds, even eight hours after a big anthocyanin dose. I made efforts to promote the control drink as equally good for her memory, but maybe she wasn't fooled. I tried to keep my tone and manner the same on testing days with or without the control, but one's own child might well see through the act. Unlike in Williams's controlled study, I didn't make sure the other foods she ate were identical on both testing days. There's also the possibility that she taught herself how to game the RAVLT a little. She told me she wasn't putting as much effort into remembering the B list. Perhaps she could retain more A-list words because she tuned out the B list.

But I couldn't deny that she had held up her end of the deal. I had promised chocolate as a reward for all the testing.

"What about my treat?" she asks, eagerness and reproach on her face. "It's the right thing to do, Mama."

"What?"

"Keep your word."

"Of course."

That she remembers.

III

Body Changes Mind

JULY

Uneven Playing Fields

Can movement help kids juggle more in their minds?

WE ARRIVE IN Vermont in the thick of summer, fields all gold and green, red clover and foxglove. UJ bounds out of the car, where she sat for six hours in quiet misery. *Free at last, free at last!* The moment Ami's little silver shoes hit the grass, she too is off, shrieking in ecstasy. It's a photographic moment if I've ever seen one, and I fail to capture it because I'm standing in my city wedges, looking out, dumbstruck. Here we are in the great outdoors: dappled sunlight, a semimowed meadow, low flocculent clouds lying over a one-hundred-eighty-degree view of mountains. And down in a valley below our rental cabin, a stream-fed pond.

The next morning, UJ and I rush downhill to that stream. We take off our shoes; our feet are white, almost transparent, suety and tender. Step-by-step we plod upstream, navigating through the muck and slime, the stabby little rocks, the knifelike blades of grass along the edges. The first half hour is all sharp pain and soft fascination: "Look, a water strider! Mama! The water looks like velvet flowing over that stone!"

"You'll get a Native American sole by the end of the month," I say in a joking singsong.

It's a good time until, abruptly, it's not. "Mama! Oh no!" UJ lifts her pale, dripping foot out of the mud and almost knocks me over with it.

"Mama?" she says. "Is that a leech?"

She leans on me as I twist her foot around and pry her toes open. Attached to the pink webbing between her middle toes is what appears to be a new brownish-green toe.

I pinch the sucker and pull it off. There's blood, and it's not the leech's.

"Wow! Look at that little guy go!" I chuckle affectionately as I toss the parasite back in the stream. UJ will turn six this month. This is an impressionable age, and I desperately want her to love nature, not fear it.

The child looks at me and smiles the most ingenuous, beatific smile. I think my heart will break.

"My first leech!"

Ah, summer, what power you have to make us suffer and like it.
—Russell Baker

I have something else riding on the city kid's willingness to go shoeless. My focus this summer is on active proprioceptive exercise. Think of an old-fashioned childhood summer activity and it's likely to qualify. Navigating uneven terrain with bare feet is proprioceptive. Climbing a tree is proprioceptive. Balancing, arms outstretched, while walking on a log is proprioceptive, and so is navigating over, under, and around obstacles. Climbing over stuff soldier-style, with a sack or a big stick over one shoulder, is classically proprioceptive. Do any of the above exercises without footwear and you get extra proprioceptive points—especially if the foot strikes the ground in the middle or at the toes, not the heel. This apparently leads to greater sensory feedback to the nervous system.

The word *proprioception* comes from the Latin *proprius* ("one's own") and *capere* ("to take or grasp"); it means to have a sense of one's own body as it moves. A proprioceptive activity stimulates the system of receptor nerves (proprioceptors) located in the muscles, joints, and ligaments. Proprioceptive tasks require you to sense your position in space on a totally subconscious level. It's a sort of sixth sense.

Returning to the creek after getting bled by a leech is like getting back in the saddle after being bucked off a horse. For psychological and proprioceptive purposes, we return the next day, and tragedy nearly strikes again. Something gives way under UJ's foot, and she begins to fall. Prehensile instinct kicks in, and her right hand shoots out and grabs (grasps) a rock that juts out of the water. Restabilized! There's a wobbly smile on her face. Then she takes two steps, the liquid-gold water lapping at her knees, and slips again, this time gashing her leg on a rock. She's down, then up, wet, her face bright red under the blazing sun. Each step is different: muck, rock, oozy, sharp, rough. Right foot, left foot, sometimes rhythmic, often not.

This is what I mean by proprioceptive. The body must restabilize in every instant. The instability stimulates: you're always scanning, observing, absorbing, acting, reacting. In the midst of uncertainty, the mind is busy. It reminds me of dodging and weaving on a bicycle through Manhattan traffic. The mind must be entirely present, or else. It's almost a meditation.

The brain is like a muscle. When we think well, we feel good.
—*Carl Sagan*

Proprioceptive exercise recruits the two major brain domains: the cerebrum, Latin for "brain," and the cerebellum, the "little brain" located right under the cerebrum and on top of the spinal cord. For generations, the cerebrum was the hallowed "thinking brain" while the cerebellum was dismissed as "reptilian" neural matter. The cerebellum, it was thought, just coordinates humdrum activities such as motor control, breathing, balance, and posture. It keeps us balanced and blinking. The "little" brain represents only 10 percent of the brain's volume but contains 50 percent of the brain's total neurons (85 billion neurons, that is), which, if you think about it, suggests a suspiciously high level of brainpower for blinking and mouth breathing. But all but a few visionary types pooh-poohed the possibility that the reptilian brain could do anything interesting. Surely, it couldn't do anything *cerebral.*

Now that old way of thinking is getting turned on its head. There's a quiet movement—the dawn of a "cerebellar epoque"—thanks to advances in medical imaging and computational modeling. In the past fifteen years, more than two hundred studies have revealed that the cerebellum is active during tasks that don't involve movement at all. It plays a mysterious role in purely cognitive tasks. There's even evidence that pathways go from the prefrontal cortex in the cerebrum—the thinking and planning part of the brain—to the cerebellum, where the information is processed and then fed back to the cerebrum.

This makes the cerebellum something of a black box, and we can only guess what's going on inside. The Harvard Medical School neurologist Jeremy Schmahmann has a theory that he calls the Universal Cerebellar Transform. The cerebellum, he says, integrates internal and external stimuli, which fine-tunes our learning and emotions just as it fine-tunes and coordinates our muscle movements. Another cerebellum expert, Larry Vandervert, believes that the cerebellum is always on in the background, silently gleaning information from the prefrontal cortex. Vandervert isn't suggesting the cerebellum is a passive learner. Rather, it helps us to predict and anticipate whatever it is we encounter next, and it sends that intel back to the prefrontal cortex. Its contribution enhances everything from planning, learning, speaking, and listening to coding and retrieving memories. Damage your cerebellum, the theory goes, and you'll have trouble thinking and remembering.

With this understanding, the old divide between movement and cognition—mind and body—breaks down, and what follows is a fiery burst of questions and dreamy possibilities. If you activate the cerebellum in certain ways, do you think better and remember more?

There's a lot of leg work to do.

Working memory even beats IQ at its own game. . . . [It] is 3 to 4 times more accurate than IQ in predicting grades in spelling, reading, and math. —Ross and Tracy Alloway

Enter the Alloways, Ross and Tracy, a husband-and-wife team at the University of North Florida. Tracy is a psychologist and Ross is a neuroscience researcher. The Alloways' focus is on proprioceptive exercises as they apply to working memory, which is the ability to hold and manipulate several pieces of information in real time.

It's worth thinking about what working memory makes possible. The Alloways compare it to a mental work space or scratch pad because it allows us to focus on, process, and juggle information for a task at hand. We need working memory when we're visualizing how to rearrange the furniture in the room, literally or figuratively. We rely on working memory in the time span between hearing a phone number and dialing it, or when adding up the cost of groceries in our heads. Multitasking—say, juggling a Twitter feed and a text message dialogue while talking on the phone—requires formidable working memory skills. I'm taxing my working memory by organizing this chapter in my mind before I write it, and you need working memory to follow this chapter's thread back to where it began with the cerebrum-cerebellum connection and the examples of proprioceptive exercises.

Working memory is not short-term memory. You use short-term memory when you find your way to the house on Blueberry Street (left on Currant, sharp left at the fork onto Blackberry Lane; another right up the hill to Aubergine, then straight until you reach Boysenberry Bakery, where you'll take a hairpin right turn). To get back, you need to draw on your short-term memory to get the original directions, then use working memory to reverse them, turn by turn.

If you assume that working memory's primary engine is the hippocampus, where memory is stored, you'd be wrong. It's the prefrontal cortex, which is why if your hippocampus is ever damaged you'd still be able to have a running dialogue with a person you just met—working memory's scratch pad still works—but if she leaves the room and returns a minute later, you wouldn't remember her or what you'd been talking about. Normally, when you're done manipulating information on your mental scratch pad, you might send it back to your short-term memory. If it's something you need to remember much later, or that you've learned repeatedly, you'd store it in your long-term memory.

For years Tracy Alloway tracked the working memory of a group of kids, from kindergarten to sixth grade. Some had poor working memory: They struggled to recall a string of digits or words either forward or backward. They'd fumble when trying to follow instructions, space out on the details of what they were doing, or lose their place while working through a complicated task. (About 10 to 15 percent of schoolchildren have working memory problems, but most parents don't know it.) Alloway and her colleagues tested the kids for working memory, as well as reading and math skills, at five, then waited two years and tested the kids again. Two years later, she tested them a third time, and then she tested them a fourth time at age eleven.

One afternoon, I take a page from Alloway's working memory playbook.

"Recite these numbers back to me," I instruct UJ. "5-7-9-2-9." She and I have just come back from another creek walk. She's flushed from exertion, and there's no air-conditioning in our cabin on the grassy hill. Not the best time for a memory test, perhaps, but such is the nature of field research.

The kid gives me an eyeroll. "5-7-9-2-9." Alloway could expect most children kindergarten age and up to remember a span of four or five numbers in forward order. This is just a warm up.

"Now, how about 3-9-8 *backward*?" I chirp. This is the Backward Digit Recall test that Alloway used. While reciting numbers forward is a good test of short-term memory, reciting the numbers backward is a better test of working memory because it draws on the ability to manipulate and process the information at the same time. In the study, each child was told to recall a sequence of spoken numbers in the reverse order, beginning with two numbers and increasing by one number for each level until he or she failed to recount a number in the correct order four times.

"Easy peasy!" UJ says.

"If you know it, show it," I say. I'm pretty sure she forgot the question, so I repeat it. "What's 3-9-8 backward?"

"8-9-3," she says. Bingo.

"How about 8-4-2-5?"

More than half of six-year-olds can recite three digits backward, but only 11 percent of them can remember four digits. More than half of nine-year-olds can recall four digits in reverse. More than half of fifteen-year-olds can recall five digits backward. In young kids, the prefrontal cortex is undeveloped, which is why juggling more than a few digits is so hard. It's also why children so often lose their train of thought. Working memory gets stronger throughout one's teens and twenties.

UJ pauses. Reciting four digits backward is as challenging as a backward roll up a hill. When neuroscientists use fMRI on people doing this sort of problem in real time, they see evidence of that feedback loop between the cerebellum and the prefrontal cortex.

"5-2-4-8!" UJ says, and beams. Pleased with her success, she doesn't want to ruin it with another problem. I pitch her another four digits to reverse, and she transposes two numbers then falters. This happens more than once. It's incredibly taxing for a kid younger than nine to remember four digits in reverse. Other classic ways to test working memory are spelling the word *world* backward or counting backward by sevens. (The faster one computes, without fingers, the better.)

Alloway's working memory research yielded some surprises. You might think that when it comes to the ability to read and do math, IQ scores would be more predictive of future academic success than, say, the ability to repeat digits backward or remember a sequence of colors. That wasn't the case. A child's working memory in kindergarten, Alloway found, is a stronger predictor of academic success at age eleven than intelligence. That said, gifted kids often have stronger working memories than their same-age peers—there's no doubt that it helps learning—but not always. Child prodigies almost always have prodigious working memory, but their IQ scores often aren't much higher than average. The children who struggled the most with the Backward Digit Recall test were more likely to be forgetful and easily distracted, to have less of what experts call executive function. They were likelier to make careless errors in writing and math than kids with average working memories. If you asked them to take off their shoes, stow their backpack in a cubby, turn their name tag around, and grab some crayons, they'd probably forget one or more of those steps or freeze halfway through.

Tracy Alloway also found a connection between working memory and emotional resilience. In her study of two thousand people from teens to seventy-year-olds, those endowed with the strongest working memory were also likeliest to be the most positive and optimistic. Alloway's explanation is that negative thoughts are intrusive thoughts, and it takes working memory to counter them or rechannel them positively. To bounce back from a bad thought, you need to keep a goal in mind while juggling other perhaps conflicting ideas in your head as well.

Research at Duke University, using MRI brain scans, supports the idea that working memory and emotion regulation overlap: people who showed more prefrontal cortex activity in a working memory test also had a greater ability to moderate their feelings and recalibrate their inner state. Meanwhile, in Alloway's study, people of all ages with the weakest working memory were prone to agree with pitiable statements, such as "I rarely count on good things to happen to me" or "If something can go wrong for me, it will."

This isn't as depressingly predetermined as it sounds. That's because anyone, at any age, can boost their working memory. It's the most heartening discovery. Unlike IQ, which seems more or less fixed, working memory is not dependent on socioeconomic background or prior education. It naturally gets stronger with age, until one's thirties.

"If your child is older, don't worry: you didn't miss the boat," Ross Alloway says, which is a relief to parents (like me) who always think they overlooked something crucial and irrecoverable in their child's early development that would have made all the difference had they only *known*. With strategic effort, a weak working memory today can become a muscular working memory tomorrow.

Which spins us back, full circle, to proprioception.

If it doesn't challenge you, it doesn't change you. —Fred Devito

Many years ago, when Tracy and Ross Alloway lived in Scotland, they picked up an eccentric local habit: barefoot running. As they jogged side-by-side without foot protection in the rocky Highlands they realized that they didn't chat with each other as they did when jogging on the street. Their minds didn't wander. That's because they knew if they took one false step their feet would be wet, muddy, bleeding, or deep in dung. They also noticed that although their barefoot workouts thoroughly taxed their attention and information-processing abilities, they didn't crash at the end of a run. Instead, they felt much sharper and clearer.

Studies have long shown that when, say, a septuagenarian spends time every day on a balance beam or navigates an obstacle course, he or she becomes more flexible physically. What's often overlooked is that he or she will also score better on a test that requires mental agility, the ability to plan ahead or put together pieces of information or draw on a memory. Perhaps, the Alloways thought, our bodies become less flexible when the mind's proprioceptive capacities wane. And vice versa: maybe our minds become less flexible as we lose that loose-limbed ability to duck and swerve and clamber and stay steady while foraging through an ever-changing context.

To test a connection between working memory and proprioceptive exercises, the Alloways recruited adults across a wide age range, divided them into an experimental group and two control groups, and tested their baseline working memory. The experimental group completed two sessions of dynamic proprioceptive exercises: the first for two hours, the second for two and a half. They climbed trees, worked their way along a three-inch wide beam, crawled forward and backward, navigated obstacles, and lifted and carried bulky objects. They tried to master a guerrilla-style technique of jumping and landing on the ball of the foot with bent knees. These exercises fall under the umbra of activities that our ancient ancestors (and my toddler) engaged in daily. The control groups, meanwhile, practiced yoga or listened to a lecture.

The Alloways gave everyone in the study a backward digit recall test after each session. All participants started at around the same degree of competence in remembering three, four, or five digits backward. But here's the striking news. Even after the first of the two exercise sessions, the proprioceptive group scored not just better but a dramatic *50 percent* higher on working memory tests than the other groups.

But heck! Who, since our hunter-gatherer days, has two hours a day for climbing trees and clambering around with sticks on their shoulders? (Even 25 percent of kids these days have never climbed a tree in their lives.) The Alloways, perhaps sensing that this was fantastical, launched a follow-up study that looked into how quickly and easily a working memory boost could be achieved. This time they simply asked adults to run barefoot on a track and jump on targets (to simulate the proprioceptive qualities of an outdoor barefoot run where you'd have to navigate around objects in the path).

Sixteen minutes of barefoot running, the Alloways found, led to a 16 percent working memory boost compared to the same run while wearing sneakers or when running barefoot on flat surfaces without targets. In theory, a 16 percent boost in working memory might make all the difference between, say, remembering an instruction or forgetting it, being derailed in the middle of a thought or calculation, or not. Best of all, sixteen minutes is doable.

I should mention that any sort of aerobic activity is good for memory because it increases blood flow to the brain. Vigorous exercise raises brain-derived neurotrophic factor (BDNF), a chemical that triggers the growth of extra neurons in the hippocampus, the area of the brain critical for learning and memory. Harvard researchers found that two hours of any regular heart-pumping aerobic exercise a week increases the size of the hippocampus within six months.

But the exercises the Alloways prescribe have two criteria: first, they're proprioceptive; and second, they include locomotion or navigation as the environment or terrain changes. The combination, they say, is the key to a working memory boost instead of only a boost to the hippocampus where memory is stored. Think about it: to navigate uneven, springy, jungly terrain while awkward, encumbered, and sneakerless is a whole-brain workout. If you're barefoot jogging, you have aerobic activity combined with sensory input from the sole of the foot, striking the ground from the ball to toe, combined with the uneven pacing and just-in-time route planning to avoid injuring the foot. You have body awareness *plus* mindful movement. Yoga poses may be proprioceptive but they're too static, which is why they failed to improve working memory. (Yoga practices that involve more dynamic movement may yield different results.)

The whole-brain workout—proprioception plus movement— draws more on the prefrontal cortex than regular aerobic exercise does, and it's the prefrontal cortex that coordinates working memory, explains Ross Alloway. Brain scans also show that when working memory is taxed, the cerebellum is more active, even when a person isn't moving, so there's a surefire connection there as well.

The hot question is whether this sort of cerebellar workout transfers to broader skills like mental rehearsal, the ability to visualize or create an event in one's mind. Larry Vandervert and others have suggested that it just might. The cerebellum—with practice and experience— learns to predict not only, say, where a moving ball or body part will be in space and time but also cognitive processes like the speed and consistency of words or speech. What may be happening in the mysterious black box of the cerebellum is a mechanism that anticipates or "rehearses" what's next and feeds that signal back to consciousness in the prefrontal cortex. The cerebellum might also help us to suspend information while we do the mental maneuvering, or speed it up so that we can do math or reverse directions or do the backward recall test or anything else that requires us to juggle the various parts of an operation. The better this circuit works, the stronger the working memory.

On these soft, glowing midsummer afternoons I establish a half-hour workout for UJ and myself, although that noun sounds wrong. If our new exercise routine had to be defined, it would be closer to natural movement, which is a regimen based on the way our ancestors navigated around ditches and gullies and other rough terrain. Another term that comes to mind is *parkour*, a movement routine based on military obstacle course training. Both evoke the return of, or a celebration of, the native or the warrior.

Biohack: Go Proprio

Any type of physical fitness translates into cognitive benefits, but proprioceptive exercise—a.k.a. "the way our ancestors moved"—may be the best for a working memory boost. The Alloways' experiments involved a series of three- to five-minute exercises that include two criteria: proprioception (positioning, balancing, and orienting the body) along with locomotion or navigation (movement). Some of the exercises in their experiments include:

- crawling forward, backward, and laterally, with the right hand and left foot in motion while the left hand and right foot stay on the ground, and vice versa
- navigating over and under 3-foot-high bars
- moving from a squatting to standing position
- running barefoot and focusing on landing on the ball of the foot with bent knee

- carrying a weight on the left or right shoulder while relaxing the opposite side

Natural movement and parkour introduce an array of other options, all appealing to Navy SEALs and the under-thirteen set:

- climb up onto a tree branch from a bat-hang position
- leap over logs, jump from big rocks, or run at them at top speed and bound off them
- crab crawl (legs wide, chest upward, butt high)
- monkey walk (legs spread wide, butt low)
- get up from the floor without using your hands (over and over again)
- climb a fence, climbing wall, pile of rocks, or other structure

All these exercises require a person to strategize different ways that the exercise can be done. Challenge the kid. *What's the most efficient way you can do it?* (Brainstorm.) *How quickly can you do it?* (Time them.) *How many times in a row can you do it?* (Count it, gameify it.)

For the city kid, try swimming in an indoor pool, walking on all fours in a big room, jumping, balancing, and defending an object. Ross Alloway recommends a school track or blacktop. Tell the kids to peel off their shoes and socks and run barefoot around the circle, picking up sticks or other objects as they go—a variation of the proprioceptive dynamic exercise in his working memory study. Just fifteen minutes can have a great impact, he says.

To give your kid the Backward Digit Recall test for working memory, simply read a series of numbers out loud, then ask him or her to recall them to you in reverse order (2-4-6-7 in reverse is 7-6-4-2). This test is also used to strengthen working memory. While my focus was on strengthening working memory with physical exercise, there are other workouts for working memory in general: for instance, card games, and the n-back test (which involves seeing a string of digits and recalling what number appeared two, three, four, or more digits earlier in the sequence). There's also some evidence that "talking" with hands helps to improve working memory when doing math or describing an experience.

(Note: the movement exercises in the Alloways' study were designed by MovNat, a fitness education system, although the researchers are not financially connected to MovNat.)

UJ's appearance has taken a feral turn this summer. Her skin is tan, nicked, scratched, and bug-bitten; there's grass in her tawny hair; and she just lost her first tooth. In the city, I'm always dragging her behind me, but here in hill country she's taken the lead. Every so often she turns around and levels me with a challenging gaze.

"Mama, come!"

Still barefoot, she clambers up rocks. She might kick the old green ball with the little nubs, the same one I used to motivate her to move as a baby, up the hill and down again. One time Ami squeals when the ball rolls downhill, so UJ keeps kicking it, laughing savagely, until it rolls into the creek. She ducks through the underbrush, saves the ball heroically from a mud trap in the water, then carries it back up through the dewy ferns. "Do it again!" I shout. "And again! Run up the bumpy hills and roll down. Drag a branch! Run up again, and this time try to somersault down! Hotdog-roll down! Kick the tires on the car each time you run around the house barefoot, and I'll count the seconds." I must sound like a drill sergeant.

Meanwhile, eighteen-month-old Ami lumbers after us, arms out-stretched, shrieking with delight. The cerebellum grows by an astounding 240 percent in the first year of life, laying the groundwork for a child's central executive and working memory. (There is a need for research on the impact of motor activity on the development of working memory.) We all move like shadows as the sunlight drifts into the copper of early evening. There's a skitter of crickets in the grass.

"Mama, my feet hurt!" UJ finally says.

"Your soles still aren't tough enough!"

Our romps amid the greenery have a timeless quality. We're hot and uncivilized. We have the right spirit, if not perfect form.

What have I noticed after these workouts? For one, a state of heightened alertness that Ross and Tracy Alloway had observed in themselves in the Scottish Highlands. In the spirit of fun, we try the Backward Digit Recall test before and after a proprioceptive workout. Afterward, UJ turns the digits around quickly, with greater speed or gusto than usual. Five digits are out of reach, but three are easy and she can even do four sometimes. When she falters, she shrugs more often than she tantrums, and more frequently tries again. If there's overlap in the circuits of working memory and emotional regulation, strengthening the former may be helping the latter.

But if there's any consistent, quirky, and unexpected cognitive benefit that I've observed, it's her speech. Like most kids, and some adults, UJ often speaks haltingly. She might start a sentence then pause, start again, stop. Her thoughts unwind—sometimes woolly, sometimes refined—as if from a giant spool. There are often fillers: the grating *like*, the ubiquitous *um*, and repetitions of words and phrases. But after a half hour or longer of proprioceptive exercise, I notice that her speech is more fluid and filler-free. The words flow like a stream. When the words pour out more quickly, ideas follow. There's more—more questions, more free-range thinking, a gush of *what-if*s. It's as if a dam has burst.

Could this be real? You can argue that anything that stimulates us makes us more attentive, which in turn could improve fluidity of speech. She's on vacation. Her sixth birthday is at the end of the month, and there's a lot of anticipatory exuberance. Aerobic exertion and an increase in maternal cheerleading might also explain why she's more "on" when she's expressing herself. Perhaps the smoother speech is just an artifact of a faster heartrate, cerebral blood flow, adrenaline, endorphins, and other perks of exercise.

But there's also a case to be made that dynamic proprioceptive exercise in particular improves the fluidity of speech (as well as thought). Working memory is required when we need to speak out loud while holding in mind the thoughts that follow. This is *verbal* working memory, which involves holding, or storing, information in the mind for one to two seconds. Verbal working memory is what you need to be able to talk while thinking about or mentally rehearsing what to say next. Verbal working memory also affects the timing and rhythm of speech, maybe the extent to which we're silver-tongued. Whether stimulating the cerebellum improves verbal working memory is unknown; as usual, we need more research.

How long we can expect to savor the benefits of exercise on working memory has been hard to quantify. UJ's verbal enhancement often lasts the rest of the day but doesn't necessarily spill over to the next. But what if we kept up these workouts for weeks or months? When rodents exercise on a running wheel for nine weeks, they, like us, enjoy a lovely cognitive boost immediately afterward. But when tested for general cognitive performance two to four weeks after they stop exercising, whatever good it did is a long-distant memory. However, of note, when mice enjoy six weeks of voluntary aerobic exercise plus three additional weeks of working memory training (learning to solve mazes), they do have a longer-lasting boost in brainpower than after either activity alone. When tested up to a month after they dropped both activities, mice in this group performed over twice as well on cognitive tests as the mice who received only memory training or aerobic activity alone.

To the Alloways' point, dynamic proprioceptive exercise incorporates both working memory and physical challenge, so this type of workout may be ideal for long-term brain benefits. Ross Alloway says the accumulative benefits are still a mystery and are untested in humans, but he offers insights from his own experience. When you stop your dynamic longtime proprioceptive workouts, he says, you notice the working memory difference within days. It's not for the better.

Life is like riding a bicycle. To keep your balance, you must keep moving. —Albert Einstein

On the soft summer evening of July 22, UJ blows out six candles on a peanut-butter-chocolate-chip-cookie ice cream cake. She's light-hearted. She is wearing a new fuchsia sundress and has a view of green mountains. She reveals two of her birthday wishes. One, no more pollution. Two, to ride a two-wheeler.

I feel a kind of acceleration. Bicycling! After a month of country workouts, I have been wondering how to keep up the exercise once we go home to the city. Bike riding qualifies as somewhat proprioceptive. It requires core stability, balance, strength, endurance, and sensory feedback about position and movement of the muscles, joints, ligaments, tendons, and connective tissues. It involves movement and navigation: swerving around potholes and vertebrates wearing lizardskin Prada.

But first there's an Everest to climb. To ride a bike, she needs to learn to balance, get over the fear of falling, and get up after a crash. She'll need to keep pedaling to stay upright even when her instinct says to stop. Come to think of it, this just about sums up the challenges of the cerebellar epoque: to stay steady, steer well, and use momentum to keep moving forward.

That's my birthday wish for her.

AUGUST

The Right Touch

The cutting edge in hands-on research

T HE SKY OVER the Seventy-Sixth Street basketball court has a tender pink glow on August evenings. It's the second day we're there, and it's the same crowd: a pack of preschool boys on scooters, each with a black-and-red ninja headband wrapped around his helmet; a team of raging manboys shouting and shooting hoops; and a sporty mother-son duo. The two have set up a portable tennis net and serve each other with gladiatorial gusto.

At least they do until my daughter, unsteady on her new pink two-wheeler with handlebar tinsel, crashes right through their net with a sorrowful wail. This dynamic proprioceptive stuff—balance, coordination, strength, speed—doesn't always come easily to the child learning how to ride a bike. I grumble an apology to the mother and son and direct UJ and her bike back to the perimeter of the court.

"Pedal, pedal, pedal!" I shout, shoving her off for the umpteenth time. She pedals once, twice, spins woozily and . . . down she goes again. It's the same clattering crash every time, an explosion of tinsel everywhere, and we've clocked in over four hours already. After every wipeout she squats, put her hands on her knees, and heaves herself to her feet. She's incredibly resilient (credit the good gut microbes), but progress is elusive. After one particularly nasty spill she puts her head in her hands and a small group assembles around her. One of the little ninja guys wants to tell her that *he* can do it, and his babysitter erupts in hard, bright, careless laughter. A pint-sized brute asks *me* if he can have a turn riding my daughter's bike now. Then a tiny girl rides over, brakes her two-wheeler elegantly, and gawks at the big skinned-kneed kid on the ground. UJ scans the crowd unblinkingly, then slowly drops her head back in her hands.

Enter Ami. Little Ami in a strawberry-print shirt and matching bloomers toddles in from who-knows-where she's been with Peter and hurls herself at her big sister. Her hug is so tight that UJ would normally complain, but this time she hugs the baby back with equal force. They release one another, then hug again, even though Ami is drooling. And a third time. Then, with a little shake, UJ wipes her tears on her riding glove and gets back on the bike.

Why didn't I think of that?

When UJ was a toddler and falling constantly, I kept my face neutral (as I do now), but I'd hug her, kiss her boo-boos gently, then let her get back up again. She was delectable, squeezable, with dimpled cheeks and thighs, always scented with our favorite comfrey baby shampoo. Then, I don't know exactly when—maybe around age four-and-a-half but possibly earlier—I stopped all the hugging and kissing and cuddling every day, or even most days. Even when she'd trip on the uneven sidewalk or fall off her scooter, there were no more hugs or boo-boo kissing. Meanwhile, our physical affection is focused Ami-ward. Peter and I are always making "Ami sandwiches": squeezing her in between us, kissing her flushed cheeks, and massaging her compact toddler body. Was UJ denied the same affection when the baby arrived and became the main recipient of Mama's touch? I cannot say.

In many Western families, touch tapers off quickly. In a study that tracked physical affection throughout a child's first year of life, psychologists found that both maternal affectionate and stimulatory touch decreased markedly around the six-month mark as other expressions of affection take over. And it's true. Instead of squeezing the six-year-old and smothering her with kisses, as I do with Ami, I just compliment the kid. *Great job scraping yourself off the ground again!*

I don't speak for every parent, obviously. The extent to which moms and dads and other family members affectionately touch their bigger kids depends largely on culture. Many traditional cultures maintain continuous contact. Euro-American cultures, observed the British anthropologist Ashley Montagu, touch the least and have the most touch-related taboos. Especially in affluent circles, school-age kids and teens don't get touched often. Teachers, coaches, and babysitters may be concerned that physical affection would be interpreted the wrong way, given the horrifying reality of physical and sexual abuse. People who weren't touched a lot as kids may not be particularly touchy-feely as parents. My own family was not physically expressive with me—I was the older child "born without an umbilical cord," as Mom put it—so maybe it's no surprise that I've been more hands-off as a parent.

What if that were to change?

Touch has a memory. —John Keats

How older kids might respond to a conspicuous increase in touches and hugs and kisses depends in part on how much physical affection they received in infancy. "Touch has a memory," wrote the poet John Keats, and the earliest memories of touch register indelibly on a subconscious level. One study found that a mother's sensitivity in a baby's first six months (the number of face-to-face exchanges, cra-dling, Eskimo kisses, etc.) can predict all manner of future behavior: how well she does on cognitive tests up to age five, how he interacts with the other kids on the kindergarten playground, how well she adjusts to adolescence and copes with typical teen depression. (Of course, sensitive mothers of six-month-olds are likely to also be sensi-tive moms of sixteen-year-olds, so I'd bet there's more to credit than those early ministrations.)

As further testament to the power of touch, another study found that sustained body contact and baby massage in the first few weeks after birth can reverse the harmful effects of a stressful pregnancy on the baby. That's remarkable if you think about it. Prenatal stress, which may otherwise program a baby to be anxious and high-strung may be *reversed* by something as simple as the right touch after birth. (Must the affection come from the mother? Certainly not. It can be any warm adult attachment figure.)

We—and by we I mean all mammals—can live without seeing, without hearing, without tasting or smelling, but we cannot live well without touch. In the 1960s, psychologist Harry Harlow's experiments on monkeys proved that when you deprive babies of any physical contact, they grow up to develop severe panic disorders. Sadly, the same went for orphaned Romanian infants in the 1980s who were fed but untouched in their institutionalized cribs. Follow-ups on those children and others found that the absence of devoted acts of love— especially in the first six months of life—changed the structure and function of the brain, which leads to mental illness and an (often irreversible) inability to connect with others. A touch can become a proxy for social connectedness, which is a predictor of health and mental well-being.

In the aughts, the McGill University neuroscientist Michael Meaney revealed how and why touch in early life has a lifelong effect on the nervous system and social behavior. Experimenting on rats,

Meaney took genetically identical babies and split them into two groups: one with an affectionate mother that licked and groomed, and the other with a standoffish low-licking mother. The nurtured rats grew up to be calm adults, socially well adjusted and high lickers. The rats that grew up without maternal licking grew up to be cagey, neurotic, and high-strung (which sounds tragic until you realize that this behavior is an advantage when conditions are unpredictable and one needs to keep up one's guard). A subsequent cross-fostering experiment showed that babies born to low lickers grew up to be nurturing moms when placed with nurturing, high-licking foster moms, and vice versa.

The difference in the baby's long-term outcome, Meaney concluded, isn't dictated by the genes. It's *epigenetic*: a mother's nurturing (or lack thereof) "programs" the pups' genes to behave in a certain way, without altering the DNA itself. If you want to get technical, the physical contact activates a gene that codes for glucocorticoid receptors in the hippocampus, the brain region responsible for memory and attention. Glucocorticoid is a stress hormone, and having a lot of glucocorticoid receptors is like having a lot of smoke detectors in your house. The sooner these receptors detect the slightest whiff of cortisol and bind it, the sooner they release anti-inflammatory proteins and the faster the stress circuit shuts down—a good thing, because excess cortisol leads to neurotic, on-edge, even aggressive behavior that you often see in kids who've been deprived of physical affection. The remarkable thing is, there's nothing in the genes that determines for sure how many glucocorticoid receptors we grow. Nurture nudges that number.

Touch research also shows that when touch is happily received— it isn't always, of course, but when it is—the body's vagus nerve is activated (the same one that *Lactobacillus* and *Bifidobacterium* use to communicate with the brain), and the vagus carries the feel-good signal into the brain regions that regulate mood. Brain scans show that touch activates the orbitofrontal cortex, a part of the brain that can control feelings of reward. An affectionate touch can trigger a rise in oxytocin, the hormone that helps bonding, trust, and a sense of safety. Touch can lower blood pressure and heart rate as well as cortisol levels.

You start to see how all this leads to a big advantage when it comes to feeling a little calmer during an intense performance or other high-stakes moments. (In one experiment, women who underwent the threat of electric shock had much less cortisol when holding hands with their husbands. The closer the relationship, the lower the women's cortisol and the better their emotional regulation.) The prefrontal cortex, which had been so busy trying to stabilize wobbly unstable emotions, is free to finally focus on the situation at hand. A touch can say, *Relax. I've got your back. I see you. I understand you. You're not alone.*

Touch is ten times stronger than verbal or emotional contact, and it affects damn near everything we do. —Ashley Montagu

Not long ago, a team led by Annett Schirmer at the Max Planck Institute in Germany recruited nearly fifty five-year-olds and their mothers to participate in an experiment. First, they asked every mother-child duo to play together with some blocks as they would at home while Schirmer and her team watched. The mothers did not know it, but the researchers were counting the number of times they touched their children. The average was about one touch a minute, with some "high-touch" mothers touching more frequently and "low-touch" moms touching less or not at all. Two weeks later, the researchers asked the kids to rest in an fMRI scanner and watch a picture of a lava lamp.

Why put kids through this? Schirmer was curious about what each child's brain would look like in the resting default mode—or mind-wandering state—when they weren't engaged in a task. Would the regions linked with social cognition be active? If they were in default mode, that would suggest that the child's social brain was strong or well developed, the scientists thought, especially in the "theory of mind," which is the ability to understand that another person's beliefs, desires, perspectives, and values are different from one's own. Children with a well-developed theory of mind are better at predicting how others will react to them or to a situation. So, what's your prediction? Would the kids of high-touch moms show more activation of the social brain, even at times of rest, than the kids of low-touch moms?

If you guessed yes, you're right. The scans revealed that the more a mother had touched her child during the play observation—a "thin slice" of their relationship—the more overlap there was between that child's default mode network and his or her social brain network. This included a circuit between the prefrontal cortex and the empathy-processing insula that didn't exist in low-touched kids. Schirmer and her colleagues are careful to point out that this is correlation, not causation. Yet "one may speculate," they wrote in the study, "that children with more touch more readily engage the mentalizing component of the 'social brain' and that, perhaps, their interest in others' mental states is greater than that of children with less touch."

One more thing about the prefrontal cortex and insula: they continue to develop through adolescence. It's not too late, right?

Keeping moms happy should be a priority. —Michael Meaney

At first I try in little feints, almost shyly. When she is telling me about her dream house (hearths, hammocks, a fireman's pole that goes from an attic in the clouds to the ocean floor) I reach over and give her a bear hug and mess up her hair. She smilingly extricates herself and keeps on talking. Later, when I am cuddling with Ami, I draw her in with us. *You're loved.* She lets herself be kissed for two or three seconds, then shrieks and throws a pillow at us.

It hits me with a dull thud. It's easy to give UJ more physical affection in these times when we're relaxed, but perhaps the best way to test the power of parental touch is at a time of tension. During violin practice, for instance. I'm no Tiger Mom, but I demand focus and respect. I tell her when she's playing sloppily or if I hear a wrong note. These efforts are not met with gratitude.

An opportunity presents itself in her next violin practice. She plays a piece with the wrong ending. "Uh oh!" I say brightly. That sort of "uh oh!"—a chiding singsong—grates on her as much as an out-of-tune string instrument does to me. She looks at me sharply and in a clenched voice tells me that *she already knew that.* Then she goes back to playing and promptly makes the same mistake again. I shake my head, lips zipped. She combusts with rage and frustration.

I don't touch her shoulder in this moment. That would seem, well, heavy-handed. But I kiss her heated brow. And as I rub her back she gives a sort of rattled shake, steps back, and does something that normally takes at least five minutes after a meltdown. She turns back to her violin. The touch seems to have conveyed my intended message: I accept her, foibles and all. It communicated that I'm not harboring discontent or disappointment.

Afterward, she hugs me. Then she makes a humbling, heartbreaking request. "Mama?" she asks. "Can I hug *you* when you get mad?"

Biohack: Hugs and Nudges

How effectively can we parent through touch alone? For the month, I tried a hands-on approach to testing the science of touch. Here are the benefits based on lab-tested experiments:

- *Stress reduction*: When the child is anxious, hold hands with him for six to twelve seconds. (A study on medical patients found this simple gesture of social rapport significantly reduces anxiety.) On my kid, this gesture has variable success. When she is frustrated, she rips her hand out of mine and refuses eye contact. For us, a hug is more effective.

- *Cooperation and trust building*: A study on NBA players showed that the more teammates touched each other early in the season, the better their performance as the season unfolded. These touches included butt slapping, high fives, chest bumps, fist bumps, low fives, head grabs, full hugs, half hugs, and team huddles. In our household, butt slapping is very funny, especially when the younger daughter farts on the older one, so this one was a big success. High bonding value validated.

- *Self-esteem, stress release, risk taking, trust*: Roughhouse in the form of pillow-fighting, steamrollering, tossing a child on a bed, horse rides, wrestling, and eating them up. My kids do love it when their dad throws them around. Is this why both of them are daddy's girls? (When a kid says stop, be sure to stop.)

- *Cooperation and compliance*: Experiment with a one- to two-second tap on the shoulder or upper arm. For us, this works much of the time to gain the child's attention, especially if said child is zoning out. It helps when the child is already on the same wavelength, with the same goal. However, it doesn't work consistently when the child (or adult) is stressed or anxious, and on these occasions has even backfired.

Touch is the central medium in which the goodness of one individual can spread to another. Touch is the original contact high.
—Dacher Keltner

Third day of learning how to ride a bicycle. We're back at the basket-ball court, and there's a dreamy late-summer softness in the evening air. Ami runs around the blacktop, at one point spinning around and around in circles and into the mosh of a soccer game played by eight-year-old boys in Emirates jerseys. By now UJ can balance on the bike, which is a sort of coup, but she crashes after a few seconds because she's still not pedaling hard enough. Her temper flares and she blames me for distracting her.

Forty-five minutes pass, and the late-August air, once balmy, becomes cloyingly hot. My back is drenched under the backpack I'm wearing. I had told UJ to keep a rhythm—*I think I can, I think I can,* anything—and keep pedaling, but she is not following directions. I find myself getting hotter, frustrated, miffed.

"Why aren't you pedaling harder? You're freezing! Don't freeze!"

"I'm not!"

"You are!" I'm ready to call it a night. I'm thirsty. "Let's do this again tomorrow," I say gently. I compliment her progress and tell her how proud I am that she balanced for a few seconds on her own. To my ears I sound kind and reasonable, even though my blood is boiling. Then I touch her shoulder. I rest it there for a leaden three or four seconds.

"No!" she shudders. "NO!"

Has my touch belied my light, calm voice? If I had not touched my daughter while trying to repress my anger, would she have had a better reaction to my words?

The answer depends on how effectively emotions are transmit-ted by touch alone, which was the focus of a body of research at the Berkeley Social Interaction (BSI) lab. The social psychologist Dacher

Keltner, who runs BSI, and his colleagues at DePauw University paired up 250 volunteers and gave each person one of two roles: an emotion "encoder" or an emotion "decoder." The challenge was for the encoder to try to communicate one of eight emotions (anger, fear, happiness, sadness, disgust, love, gratitude, sympathy) by touching the decoder anywhere (well, almost anywhere) on the body. The decoder, who was blindfolded, had to guess which emotion the encoder was trying to convey from all the shakes, strokes, pushes, hits, pats, slaps, hugs, and presses with different degrees of pressure.

Guess which emotions are conveyed most accurately through touch alone? The answer: anger, gratitude, love, fear, disgust, and sympathy. When men were on the receiving end of the touch by a woman, love and disgust were detected most effectively. When women were on the receiving end of a male touch, anger, gratitude, and sympathy were communicated best. When a female touched a female, the emotion transmitted with the highest accuracy was—memorably—anger (75 percent of the time, via pushes, shakes, and squeezes) followed by love (61 percent of the time, via hugs). When I'm angry or fed-up with UJ and touch her, there's a fair chance her nerve fibers pick up my frustration or fury even in the absence of other telltale signs.

Keltner's experiment sounded like fun, so UJ and I try it on a sunny morning when the bike is safely out of sight. I am the toucher, she the decoder, and then we swap roles. She loves it. In our variation (which I recommend all parents try with their kids), she wears a blindfold and I stand behind her. I channel all eight emotions, trying all of them repeatedly in different order. I replicate the angry playground grip: slightly firm, on the shoulder. I stroke her arm in sympathy. I sandwich her hand between mine in gratitude. I am surprised she doesn't pick that one up. Just three emotions come through loud and clear to her every time: anger, disgust, and—thank goodness—love.

That children are a lightning rod for their parents' emotions isn't exactly revelatory. But the idea that a brief moment of tactile contact can convey so much about intangibles like family expressivity and childhood connectedness is striking. Consider, for example, another little study by Keltner and his colleagues. The team carefully scanned pairs of photos of nearly one hundred kindergartners from the San Francisco Bay Area, one provided by the family and the other a school photo. They were looking for two things in the family snapshots, or so-called "thin slices" of the kids' lives: smiling and touch. Coders rated each photo for the warmth and quality of tactile contact: restraint, aggression, arm around the shoulder, arm link, handhold, hug, and others. Separately, they rated the quality of the child's smile in the school photo, which was taken solo and during the school day. A pattern emerged: the warmer a parent's touch in the family photo, the more genuine the kid's smile in the school photo, suggesting that the child was warmer or more expressive generally. Correlation isn't causation, of course, but the outcome adds an interesting data point.

It's worth mentioning for a moment the counterpart to the warm (often maternal) touch: the playful (often paternal) touch. By this I mean the act of wrestling children to the ground or torquing them in midair. This type of contact can be a pillow in the face. It's a body slam. It's a hectic frenzy, part cackling laughter, part hysteria. It's what Peter's doing when he takes Ami and hangs her upside down like a bat then swings her around by her armpits until they're both dizzy. ("Again! Again!" she squeals.) UJ seems to like roughhousing more now than she did when she was younger.

This type of touch—is it manhandling?—is baffling to me. I believe strongly that an adult should never force children to roughhouse, and I don't like tickling when the kid has no sense of control. I roll the kids around, pretend to bite them, and say, "BOO!" But I neither hurl nor heave.

Despite my reservations, the science here is persuasive. Rough-and-tumble sensory stimulation has multiple social and emotional benefits. Kids learn to communicate verbally and nonverbally. Roughhousing triggers the release of brain-derived neurotrophic factor (BDNF), the same neuron-building fertilizer triggered by exercise and blueberries and certain microbes, especially in areas of the brain responsible for memory and learning and language. Horseplay leads to fewer social and behavioral problems: there's a give and take. The kids learn to take risks. It's OK to be impish and cunning and out of control. They often feel happy and connected afterward. There's a touch of aggression, but it's *playful* aggression.

There's another apparent bonus here, too. Being in the air and upside down, toppled, tossed, and flung is proprioceptive. (The child needs to perceive where his or her body is in space, as well as how much pressure is on the joints during movement.) When young kids are touched during play they get a sense of a "body map." Body awareness is the foundation of a mind-body connection, which in turn leads to greater body acceptance and feeling comfortable in one's own skin. Literally and symbolically, proprioception is about balance.

Proprioception is also crucial for learning to ride a bike.

Life is like riding a bicycle. To keep your balance you must keep on moving. —Albert Einstein

Bike-riding lesson, day four. It's another humid August evening at the basketball court. UJ, armed with scuffed elbow pads, knee pads, and helmet, mounts her bike. I hover behind her. I feel her stiff, grim determination.

This day, I feel, is a chance to experiment with another type of touch, the coercive touch. I've used affectionate touches, angry touches, inadvertent disgust touches, playful touches. But coercive touch? Touch a person briefly, the research shows, and the touchee is more open and compliant. Sounds good to me.

The body of research on coercive touch is more than twenty years old, and it's robust. Touch a stranger on the forearm for two seconds when you're asking for help picking up stuff that you dropped, as volunteers did in a French study, and you're likelier to get a helping hand (90 percent of passersby complied versus 63 percent). Other field experiments showed that when a woman touched another woman when asking for a cigarette she was likelier to get a light. When men ask a woman for her phone number, they're likelier to get it if the request is paired with a light touch on the arm. Passersby are even likelier to agree to watch a massive dog if the owner utilizes the same light touch. Compliant touch has been replicated in many different cultures, all with the same striking results.

Children are receptive to it, too. In a classroom experiment staged by the French psychologist Nicolas Guéguen, a teacher circled around the room, leaning over his pupils' shoulders to check their work on a math problem. "Good start! That's good; you understood it!" he told them. In a low voice so that no one else could hear, he told each kid, "That's good. Well done!" Then, before moving on, the teacher gave a slight one-second tap on the upper arm to randomly selected kids.

The difference in performance between the touched and untouched groups was dramatic. Boys were nearly three times as likely to volunteer to go to the blackboard after the touch, and girls were more than four times as likely to go to the front of the room. To demonstrate how they did the math!

Recently, research on coercive touch in kids has extended into a red-hot zone: the delay of gratification. Much of the work with kids in this field has focused on variations of the classic marshmallow test, which measures impulse control and self-regulation and is thought to be predictive of academic success, standardized test scores, and social skills. A young child is given a choice: eat one marshmallow now or resist the temptation for a few minutes and get two marshmallows. Kids try every trick to prevent themselves from caving in: they chew on their lips, they put their hands under their butts, they sing "Twinkle, Twinkle Little Star" to themselves. Intriguing, right? So what would happen if you told the kid to wait before eating the candy—and then touched his or her back briefly?

A group studying touch at Wesleyan University staged this very experiment with forty four- and five-year-olds and a bag of candy. The experimenter told each kid that she hid five candies under a cup and to wait until she said it was OK to find and eat the treats. She'd leave the room, she said, but she'd be back in ten minutes. With that, she gave half the children a brief, friendly touch on the back and left. The kids found themselves alone with a cup under which they knew there was candy that must not be consumed.

Silence.

Did the kids who were touched hold out longer before looking for the sweets? Yes, it turns out, and not just a little longer, but two minutes longer on average—no doubt an eternity in the mind of a five-year-old candy lover. This was a positive sign that touching a child (on the shoulder) helps his or her ability to self-regulate. But why? In the experiment, it could have been that the touch alleviated the stress and anxiety of waiting alone in a room, the researchers theorized. Or maybe the touch made the kid feel more emotionally attached to the experimenter and therefore likelier to comply with her request. Kids are more cooperative with adults with whom they have a rapport. In any event, the touch helped the kids cope with their situation. If touch fosters self-control, the researchers concluded, then there are clear long-term benefits.

If I were to ask UJ to practice self-control or cooperation, she'd fight it. If I said *Calm down and listen*, those words would likely fall on deaf ears, or she'd turn her head. No matter how wise my counsel, she'd resist. She wants control and shuns external reinforcement. *Shhhh, Mama.* I've come to think of coercive touch as an under-the-radar influence without the pushback that comes with heavy-handed requests. That's what makes it a compelling tool for parents. *Please help set the table* (touch). *It's time to put your shoes on* (touch). *Please pay attention to the speaker* (touch). I've tried it, and it works, at least much of the time. Such a touch from a teacher or any other adult authority who is not the parent would likely lead to even higher compliance. I'd say the coercive touch boosts amenability up from 50 percent to 70 percent in our household. Which can be meaningful.

These successes inspired me to try a little field experiment at the basketball court. I want to convey to UJ my wish for her to keep it together enough to focus on pedaling her bicycle in the face of uncertainty. She must pedal through her fear about staying balanced and keep pedaling even as she wobbles. My hypothesis is that a touch from me might help her be more mentally balanced, so she won't panic and topple. Who knows, maybe the touch will reduce stress in a way that offsets my bossy verbal instructions or helps her pay more attention to them. Perhaps it will speak louder than my words.

"Pay attention to your pedaling this time," I say to UJ in a low, even voice. "Don't let yourself freeze. Keep those legs moving." I touch her lightly on the upper arm, for just a second, below her T-shirt sleeve and above her elbow pads. She's half smiling, semitentative. Then I give her seat a little shove and let go.

This time, she pedals with merciless force. "She's pedaling, still pedaling, she's pedaling!" And in no time at all she's far beyond my reach.

SEPTEMBER

99 Percent Perspiration

Using body cues for peak performance

I**T'S THE FIRST** day back to school. Outside the brick building, you can smell excitement, tension, and panic in the air. The kids are bright and brittle, including UJ, who's a little nervous because she's going to take the bus home by herself for the first time. Inside the school, on the way to her new first-grade classroom, are trophy cases: chess trophies, debate trophies, and so on. Shrines to the pointy-headed golden gods. Back in kindergarten, UJ had taken me by the hand to one of the displays and pointed.

"Look!" she whispered conspiratorially. She stood there for a few minutes gazing at the trophies in mute reverence.

My daughter's school, like many, encourages competition. The teachers no doubt see it as a friendly and benign sort of rivalry, a way to sharpen the mind and stoke the flame. So it was no surprise last school year when my trophy-dazzled daughter asked to participate in a school chess tournament. I said OK, although I worried that the competition would get in the way of her enjoyment of the game. On the day of the match I decided to be cool and not hang out or hover. At pickup time, however, I could tell that something was off.

"How was it?" I asked.

"Great," she said flatly. She was clutching a blue knight key ring, a consolation prize for students who won only one match. I looked around at the faces of other five- and six-year-olds who were also holding blue knights, and I detected distress.

"I lost two times," UJ said. Again, the monotone. The sullen face.

"Tough competition?" I asked.

"I'll tell you later," she hissed in my ear.

Outside the school, the story rushed out. A lot of kids were serious. Some were really nervous. They all wanted to win a trophy, UJ included. In the beginning of the tournament she told herself to be supercalm and superfocused; to ignore everything but the chessboard.

Then the worst thing ever happened.

She had a little accident.

She was wearing her favorite poufy, glittery butterfly skirt and thick black leggings under it, which offered protection, but she was mortified. Maybe there was a wet spot, she thought, a worry that occupied her for the rest of the tournament.

Hearing this, I had two thoughts. First, that performance pressure, especially in early childhood, must be introduced in small homeopathic doses. Even young kids whom you'd think would be oblivious, or might not seem anxious, can get apprehensive before ballet recitals or struggle under the pressure to solve a math problem in front of the class.

That led me to my second thought: I hadn't prepared my kid for performance pressure. What a gift it would be, I thought, to know how to deal effectively with this type of anxiety now, while young.

That UJ lost touch with her bladder during the chess match suggested a mind-body disconnect. One well-researched way to short-circuit the stress response—call it a hack, if you will—is to strengthen the mind-body connection. Encourage children to be more in touch with their feelings and how those feelings affect their bodies. Then guide them to use bodily cues to counteract mental stress. Instead of thinking of the body as a fleshy, leaky appendage that hampers the mind or betrays its anxiety, they can see it as a means to sharpen the mind and reduce anxiety. Instead of blocking out the signals, they can tune in to them. Tune in to their own, and even tune in to everyone else's. As it turns out, there are two interesting research-based strategies to tune in to here.

UJ, even without the poufy butterfly skirt, *you're covered.*

When your heart is already racing, you can use that high arousal in a positive way by being energetic, enthusiastic, and passionate.
—Alison Wood Brooks

Telling a child that she seems stressed doesn't always go over well. Directness can lead to denial. Or a shutdown. So, before I leave UJ to her own devices on this first day of school, I talk about what "a kid" might do *if* she were anxious about taking the bus home alone. She should home in to her own nervous energy, I say. She should feel her heart pumping wildly. She should feel the butterflies hatch in her stomach. She needs to be aware of the patina of sweat on her brow and the clammy hands. There's a technical term for what's going on, *arousal*, and it's the body's way of mobilizing resources to meet the demands of a task.

"Arousal?" UJ doesn't know the word. I tell her it means excitement.

Technically, arousal is the work of the three grand glands that make up the HPA axis (hypothalamus-pituitary-adrenal). The signal starts in the brain's hypothalamus and travels to the pea-shaped pituitary gland, which sits under it; and then it goes, via the blood-stream, to the kidney region, where the adrenals sit and churn out the hormone cortisol, which makes skin sweat and the heart beat faster. Detecting cortisol, the amygdala starts assigning emotion to experience. The usual translation is *I'm nervous!* This is how a bodily state becomes a psychological state.

What if the child can learn to make arousal work in her favor?

When I told UJ that arousal means excitement, I wasn't misleading her. But arousal can actually translate into more than one emotional state. When toddler Ami is being chased, she alternates between fear and elation, and the two emotions are almost interchangeable. She's so terrified that she doesn't want to miss a moment of it. In the same way, a new school of thought goes, if kids (and their parents) could learn to give a different label to stomach-lurching performance anxiety—*excitement* instead of, or as well as, nervousness—they'd be the stronger for it. Psychologists call this cognitive reappraisal, and dozens of studies vouch for its power and effectiveness.

Consider this classic cognitive reappraisal experiment. Students are gearing up to take a math test, and it's not just any test—it's a high-stakes standardized test with serious consequences. A few years ago, a research team made up of psychologists from Stanford, San Jose State, and the University of Denver recruited sixty students who were about to take the GRE, the standardized test to get into graduate school, and split them into two groups. Each student was given a practice exam and a note that said it's normal for people to feel anxious during standardized tests and that their hormones (via saliva) would be tested. Students in the cognitive reappraisal group also received the following note attached to their exam: "People think that feeling anxious while taking standardized tests will make them do poorly on the test. However, recent research suggests that arousal doesn't hurt performance on these tests and can even help performance. . . . People who feel anxious on the test might even do better. . . . If you feel anxious, simply remind yourself that your arousal would be help-ing you do well."

It's an interesting setup. You've got one group of students who were made aware that performance anxiety is normal, and that's that. Then you have another group that was told that if they basi-cally embraced the anxiety and rode the worry wave like a surfer, it would help them perform better.

So, how did the two groups fare? The results were so surprising that the researchers reran the numbers just to make sure they were solid (they were). First off, the cognitive appraisal group showed sig-nificantly higher levels of sympathetic nervous activity (more cortisol stress reactivity) than the control group, even though both groups were the same before taking the test. That is, when people told them-selves the stress would help them, they showed *more* physiological signs of stress, not less. On the surface, this doesn't seem like a good thing. High sympathetic nervous activity is the opposite of emotional regulation.

The amazing part was that in this case, it helped. All that nervous activity, once mentally reframed as excitement, and sustained for a short period of time, appeared to boost the students' math perfor-mance, both on the practice test in the lab and soon afterward on the actual GRE. These test-takers not only rode the worry wave, they made it swell. In fact, the actual GRE math scores between the two groups were staggeringly different: an average of 770 out of a perfect 800 for the reappraisal group versus 706 for controls. The higher-scoring group deliberately told themselves that their jitters helped their performance and they thought their nervousness helped them. When the study was published, the authors, inspired (and with a self-help angle clearly in mind), titled it "Turning the Knots in Your Stomachs into Bows."

In this context, I think maybe I shouldn't always tell my daughter to calm down when she seems jumpy and tense before a performance, even if it's something such as making an entrance at an intimidatingly large birthday party. But that's what most of us do. *Kill the butterflies. Get a grip. Don't worry. Keep calm and carry on.* In the context of performance anxiety, the "calm down" approach can even backfire dramatically.

In 1908 two psychologists, Robert Yerkes and John Dodson, developed a theorem that shows that performance increases with physiological or mental arousal. The cortisol surge increases vigilance: it's a mind sharpener. The more arousal, the better the performance on the Yerkes-Dodson scale—until it reaches a tipping point. When arousal is *too* high, working memory suffers and performance tanks. The trick is to embrace the cortisol surge without letting it overwhelm. Label it, frame it, control it. But don't deny it.

Building on the idea of an arousal "sweet spot," Alison Wood Brooks, an assistant professor of business administration at Harvard Business School, told volunteers to make an impromptu speech or take an impromptu math-based IQ test—activities that are stressful even when there's a fair warning. She divided the volunteers into three groups and instructed the first group to put on an armor of steely serenity. Close your eyes for a minute and tell yourself "I am calm," she instructed. The second group was encouraged to say to themselves, "I'm excited!" or "Try to get excited!" A third group wasn't given any instructions. As you can imagine, every heart in the room was galloping, and the only difference again was that some were told to embrace the wild ride, others were told to downgrade to a calm trot, and others were left to their own devices.

Trying to calm oneself down was indeed a bad idea. It turns out to be immensely difficult to shift from a high-arousal state (anxiety) to a low-arousal one (calm). It's like turning steam into ice. Too much mental bandwidth is spent trying to look calm and unflappable when you're feeling anything but, and it takes a toll on performance.

The superior strategy: turn steam into water vapor! That is, it's easier to shift anxiety into excitement because both are high-arousal states. The sensations of nervousness—the thumping heart, the loosening bowel—could well be exhilaration. Excitement puts us in the sweet spot of the Yerkes-Dodson scale: aroused but not overwhelmed, perfect for peak performance. As proof, the speakers in Brooks's study who were told to get excited about their butterflies were rated as more persuasive and competent, and they talked longer (a sign they were getting into it) than the other groups. Among the people who were given an IQ test, those who were told to feed their butterflies also scored higher than those in the calm and neutral conditions. They also rated themselves as more excited. They believed it.

Here, I think it's worth mentioning a problem I have with youth culture. Kids, even first graders, think that calm is always cool. Ironic detachment is *in*. The curated self, online and off, is a character that's cool and contrived. My daughter and her classmates can't really pull off "calm"—at ages six and seven, their inner fire and enthusiasm still burns (maybe too much)—but I've seen many kids just a few years older that can put on a great act. *No sweat*, but under pressure they're melting down. One in every eight children, and as many as one in five thirteen- to eighteen-year-olds, has a clinical-level anxiety disorder. Those numbers are much higher than they were in their grandparents' time. What if kids could learn to fan their enthusiasm rather than deny it?

The research shows that children six and older can reappraise negative feelings—that is, they can deliberately morph one emotion into another—but it's a skill that strengthens with age. To demonstrate, researchers at the University of Maryland used fMRI brain scans on six- to ten-year-olds as the children attempted a cognitive reappraisal exercise. When the kids reappraised a negative reaction (the mama in the photo isn't crying because she's *sad*; those are tears of *joy*!), the neuroscientists saw that the young brain grapples with the shift differently from more mature brains. In adults, the prefrontal cortex, the center of logic and reason, becomes more active during cognitive reappraisal, while the amygdala, which might assign fear to the situation, shuts down, suggesting that the prefontal cortex has the upper hand. In kids under ten years old, the prefrontal cortex is also more active as they shift from negative to positive emotions, but the amygdala doesn't shut down, which suggests that the prefrontal cortex has less sway over the amygdala and that the connection between the two regions of the brain is weaker. It's hard for researchers to read the runes: cognitive reframing for kids may take more effort, or perhaps arousal remains high enough to keep the amygdala stimulated, which isn't necessarily a bad thing when the stimulus is reframed in the positive. Later, toward the tween years and older, the prefrontal cortex has more command over the emotional amygdala.

This back-to-school month, I get a few opportunities to test cognitive appraisal on my own six-year-old. The first time I introduced the concept, she dismissed it. She had to play a violin piece in front of her classmates after a summer of lax practice. I could see her thinking about the idea of performing, then flinching away from it like a leech from salt. She said that her fingers started sweating, that they were too "juicy" to play, whatever that really means.

"So you're excited to perform in front of the group after a summer off," I said.

"No, it's just that my belly hurts."

"You're excited," I insist. "That's why your belly hurts. Flutters of excitement."

"My head hurts."

"It's bursting with excitement!"

My child looked at me in unfocused distress, arms folded, as if I were talking about her bladder.

"Just tell yourself," I said, "that all these feelings come from being excited. Not because you're nervous. OK, maybe it's a little of both, but focus on the excited part because you get to prove you can do it." I went on to explain that there's a hormone called cortisol that helps the body rise to the challenge. Cortisol feeds the butterflies and makes our hearts flutter. But it also helps us to focus and think better.

She considered this with cool amusement. "But isn't that like trying to trick myself? How can I do that?" This is the same kid that said she wouldn't fear reading the last books in the Harry Potter series because she knows Harry doesn't die; if he did, there wouldn't be more books in the series. UJ can be overly logical. And yet, she loves magic and illusion.

Distinguishing the signal from the noise requires both scientific knowledge and self-knowledge. —Nate Silver

This is what I tell her. It's a true story, and it introduces a second strategy for making performance anxiety into an advantage rather than a liability. The body's *always* tricking the brain, and the brain is always tricking the body. Tricking oneself is part of being alive, and after a while it's not a trick anymore. It's real. Plus, I say, the ways that the body tricks the brain are especially freaky and mysterious when you consider that it's not always your *own* body that can influence your brain. It can be *someone else's*. Even another kid's.

"What!"

"When people get stressed, their bodies send out mysterious signals that you take in through your nose and act on—without even realizing it," I tell her. This gets her attention because it sounds like magical Harry Potter stuff. Science, I say, can tell us a bit about these chemical signals, but there's a lot that we still don't know. We know enough to know it's not magic, even though it *seems* like magic.

"Take in through my nose?" she says, testing the phrase.

This is what we know for sure. There are two types of sweat glands. There are eccrine sweat glands, which are in the forehead, cheeks, feet, and hands. Eccrine glands produce sweat to cool our bodies down. Exercise sweat is eccrine. When we get overheated, the eccrine glands in our palms and the soles of the feet get clammy, but the sweat itself is just basically salt and water. (Stinky foot odor comes from bacteria that feed on the sweat.)

Then there are apocrine glands, which are embedded in the skin of the armpits, genital areas, eyelids, and nostrils (as well as nipples). Around age seven, eight, or nine, a kid's apocrine glands become larger and more functional. Before that age, apocrine glands are coiled under the skin, buried deep, like seeds waiting for spring. UJ is encroaching upon the years in which apocrine sweat will make its grand debut. Some of her older classmates might already be there.

Apocrine glands are more interesting than eccrine glands. Stress sweat is aprocine. Fear sweat is apocrine. Any emotional sweat, in fact, is apocrine. Apocrine glands produce a unique concoction of chemicals that includes proteins, fats, and steroids based in part on genes and in part on the status of the nervous system. Aprocrine sweat is wired to adrenaline release, which is linked with the racing heart and wobbly stomach of emotional stress . . . or excitement. It doesn't always smell pungent, but it can, and when it does it's harder to mask than eccrine sweat.

In the last few decades, a growing cadre of researchers has collected evidence and published studies suggesting that apocrine sweat contains "chemosignals" that communicate the state of a person's nervous system to all the other bodies in the area. *Pay attention! Watch me!* And even: *Watch out! Do the same!* Chemosignals can affect the behavior, emotional and hormonal states, and even the social judgments of those who breathe them.

Animals use chemosignals all the time. The dog that pees on a post is marking his territory with signals that tell other dogs to stay away. The ants at the family picnic coordinate their theft using chemosignals to communicate with one another. Many animals release chemical signals to tell others when they're in the mood to mate. The scientific case for human chemosignals includes their roles in helping newborns find a nipple; choosing and attracting partners and bonding with them; and making us feel a little more generous or fearful than we'd be otherwise. Chemosignals may also help explain why some people and places make us feel more alert or edgy.

How? The likeliest scenario is that we pick up and process chemosignals the same way we do other odors: through the main olfactory pathways. Breathe the sweat in, and a chemosensory alarm signal reaches the brain. It triggers the amygdala, the region involved in processing emotions, and the hypothalamus, which is the starting point for the production of the hormone cortisol, which, in moderate doses, stimulates us.

Think of a room, I tell UJ, where everyone is getting ready to put on a high-stakes show. Or they're about to do something daring like jump from an airplane. Or anything else that's a personal stretch. Everyone is putting out chemosignals of arousal, and it's a good thing (again, cognitive reappraisal).

"Like when riding a school bus alone for the first time?" UJ asks.

This had been a hotspot of anxiety for her in the days leading up to the first day of school. She's worried about being responsible enough to know when to get off, and if she doesn't get off at the right time and place, maybe she'll be lost on the city streets or swept away to the immense bus parking lot we once saw in the Bronx. She'd be abandoned in that cold yellow sea.

Yes, I say, riding a school bus solo for the first time is a good example. Anything that makes a person uneasy may trigger the production of chemosignals that spread the emotion to others. You can imagine that if several kids in a stuffy yellow bus are anxious, their bodies may be communicating signals that other kids detect without realizing it, and soon enough everyone's sitting a little straighter in their vinyl seat.

I had assumed that kids under seven years old surely wouldn't be able to produce chemosignals given their undeveloped apocrine glands. However, when I asked Bettina Pause, an expert on chemosignals and the chair of the biology department at Heinrich-Heine University in Germany, she argued otherwise, saying that she strongly guesses that children *do* produce these signals. In other words, don't assume that little kids can't air their anxiety. Chemosignals may be coming from their tear ducts, from the undeveloped apocrine glands, or from another body region. We need more data, but there's a lot of interesting potential there.

"So what happens if I smell sweat signals?" UJ says, wrinkling her nose and looking as if she might burst out in whinnies of laughter. It's the question on my mind, too.

Typically, in chemosignal experiments, a researcher recruits volunteers and asks them to rate their anxiety before and during a challenge. The challenge, in many cases, induces fear or anxiety: public speaking, sometimes in front of a vaguely hostile audience; scaling a tricky rope course; jumping from an airplane for the first time; or watching scary videos. All the while, the panicky or shaken-up volunteers wear collection pads in their (damp, unwashed) armpits. After an hour or two, the pads are removed, the samples pooled. The odorous mélange is thrust under the noses of oblivious volunteers. Those hapless sniffers (who know not what they're smelling) are then put through a battery of cognitive tests that assess how quickly and accurately they answer questions. Then their results are compared to those who smelled plain old exercise (eccrine) sweat from people who weren't pushed or panicked.

Is there a difference in the behavior of the anxiety-sweat sniffers versus the exercise-sweat sniffers? Yes: for one, the anxiety-sweat-sniffers are more easily startled. If the nervous system had a dial, it might go from, say, a three to a six after catching a whiff of nervous sweat. In one study using the sweat of people taking an oral exam, sniffers blinked faster after hearing an unexpected sound—the so-called startle reflex that is a test of vigilance. In another study using the armpit odors of first-time skydivers, the sniffers' brains showed increased activity in the amygdala, the area that processes emotion, and the cerebellum, which involves movement, compared to those who smelled exercise sweat.

These results suggest that the sniffers' brains were mirroring those of jittery, jacked-up skydivers. Maybe, on a biological level, this reflex coordinates group behavior. It's a signal that tells the brain that something's going on and it's better to be alert and vigilant.

It's important to note that in all the experiments the sniffers never met the donors, nor did they detect a difference between the anxiety sweat and any other sweat or substance. But their subconscious did.

Genius is one percent inspiration and ninety-nine percent perspiration. —Thomas Edison

As fascinating as chemosignals are, they wouldn't be worth mentioning here if there weren't a potential upside: better performance. We know from the cognitive reappraisal experiments that a cortisol sweet spot—heightened but not sky-high—results in better performance. Could perspiration possibly translate into secondhand inspiration?

To find out, Denise Chen, now an associate professor of neurology at Baylor University—along with her colleagues Ameeta Katdare and Nadia Lucas—did the usual rigmarole of rounding up volunteers, asking them to tuck sweat pads into their armpits, and exposing some of them to a stressor. (In this case, the group watched videos that were so terrifying or disturbing that many covered their eyes to avoid the screen.) Afterward, the research team recruited other volunteers to sniff the pads and then take a test that measured cognitive skills. How quickly and accurately, Chen wanted to know, could the stress-sweat sniffers accomplish a word association task compared to the sniffers of neutral sweat or clean, unused pads? (Note, there was no detectable difference in odor between the emotional sweat and the regular sweat.)

If you predicted that the anxiety-sweat sniffers would perform better on the tests, you're right. They were 85 percent accurate on the word association tests—more than 6 percent higher than the other groups, a statistically significant amount. (For instance, they were slightly better at identifying matches like *arms/legs* and disqualifying incongruent pairs like *arms/wind*.)

The conclusion: anxiety-sweat sniffers may have been slightly sharper in the moment. Chemosignals in the sweat primed them subconsciously to be more alert and "with it." When the test contained words that suggested a possible threat, the stress-sweat sniffers were also more cautious and took more time to respond, as if to avoid mistakes.

To the frustration of nosy parents like me, almost all human chemosensory research has been on adults only. An exception comes from the lab of Bettina Pause, the German biopsychologist, who recruited nine- to thirteen-year-old girls as her subjects. Pause and her collaborators asked the girls to smell underarm pads collected from men who had performance anxiety while taking a difficult oral exam. Later, when tested, the child stress-sweat sniffers had a swifter startle response than those who sniffed exercise sweat. Although Pause didn't give a cognitive test to the girls, she explained that a heightened startle response is a physiological indicator of alertness, which would be to a test-taker's advantage. Her study offers solid evidence that chemosignals influence children too, which opens the field to further pediatric research. (As mentioned, Pause also suspects that children emit chemosignals.)

Note that chemosignals don't *make* a person do anything. Chen and Pause, among other researchers, call the type of chemosignal in stress sweat a modulator. I call it a nudge. Exposure to the signal might tweak, enhance, or color a feeling or behavior that's already there in some measure. So if kids are in a situation in which they need to focus, like the subjects in Chen's study who were taking a cognitive test, or playing in a chess match or riding the bus home alone for the first time, the stress sweat might nudge them to be sharper and more alert. If they're in a situation in which they expect to feel vulnerable, as in Pause's startle experiment, the stress sweat might nudge them to be a little jumpier and more vigilant. If they're looking at an ambiguous unsmiling face with solemn eyes, as subjects were in another study of Chen's, the stress signal might nudge them to interpret that face as unfriendly. If people are in a relaxed mood, says Pause, the anxiety signal in stress sweat could still set them on edge but perhaps not as effectively as in a context in which they're bound to be anxious anyway.

The results from chemosignal experiments are thought-provoking. Is it really possible that something in the air—especially in the rooms where presentations and recitals, shows and exams take place—could nudge everyone to be a little sharper or perform a little better? We talk about a room's "energy" as a booster, and maybe there's more to it. Perhaps a rising tide—in this case, the SOS signal in the crowd's sweat—raises all boats. You can imagine how powerful this might be if kids use cognitive reappraisal to reframe that on-edge feeling in the body as excitement. It'd be a double boost.

As always, we need more research. No scientist has yet launched a field study to investigate whether group performance improves with the concentration of chemosignals in the room. There are so many variables: ventilation, proximity, degree of anxiety, and other forms of emotion contagion, to name a few. In the meantime, perhaps it's not a bad idea to perform (or take that standardized test) with others who are just as nervous as oneself.

Biohack: Sweat It!

On a steamy Sunday, a class of five- to nine-year-old musicians is instructed to play solos in front of a group of their peers. At least one of those children, my daughter, is rusty after the summer and, as a result, is reluctant and jittery. I can see her trepidation hours before the performance, so we try out these six research-based tricks, in hopeful anticipation that one, or some combination, or maybe just luck, will help:

- I give her the cognitive reappraisal pep talk, with directions straight out of one of the published studies. That (lurching, jittery, fluttery, sweaty, shaky) feeling, I say, is the hormone cortisol kicking in, and the cortisol will help her perform better. People who are anxious perform better. If you feel anxious, tell yourself it's helping you do better, I tell her. She thinks it's weird to try to trick herself, but I say nervousness and excitement are like two different sides of the seesaw, and she just needs to lean a little more toward the excitement side.

- I tell her to practice, for one silly minute, the superhero pose: arms extended, chin up, with an air of supreme confidence. Harvard social psychologist Amy Cuddy popularized the idea that you can "fake it till you make it." The idea is that there's a feedback loop between your actions and your mindset, so if you put on a powerful spread-limbed pose, you'll get a testosterone surge and, indeed, feel and act more powerful. While Cuddy's claim isn't undisputed, it's fun to watch my kid try to keep her chin up, in tree pose, arms extended like fairy wings. It's a distraction and makes us laugh.

- I let her sniff the black-and-white polyester blouse with the tiny flowers I wore that awful afternoon of school bus anxiety (more on this later). I tell her that the chemical alarm signals in the sweat may make her more focused. I remind her about the study in which test takers scored better after smelling the sweat of people who were scared. The sweat came from stinky armpits, and she thinks that is hilarious.

- One might argue that smelling a smelly shirt before a performance is as superstitious as it is scientific. A study at the University of Cologne suggests that activating good-luck beliefs with an action such as finger crossing or a lucky charm (clothing, ball, colors, etc.) improves performance in upcoming tasks because it helps the user feel more self-confident and persistent. Maybe, I think, my stinky panic-day shirt acts as a lucky charm. After all, science suggests it will help.

- Aerobic exercise reduces performance anxiety, so UJ does twenty jumping jacks. All the while, she is still laughing about the smelly shirt, and the effort to laugh only increases the cardiovascular effort.

- We laugh together. Who knows if any of this works, especially the stinky shirt. But what's the harm?

Within an hour, some combination of these tricks seems to genuinely improve her music performance. Maybe she was sufficiently convinced that her nervousness, or everyone else's, would nudge her into performing better. Maybe she was distracted. When it is her turn to play, my kid, dressed in her favorite tie-dye shirt, gives a great shake and raises the violin to her shoulder. She is flushed, but her tone is clean, no string crossings. She remembers the sequence of the song—a feat not consistently accomplished in the comfort of our kitchen. Whether it's the anxiety of her peers, some of them much older, or her reframing of the situation or the stinky shirt or exercises or something else altogether, it works. She pulls it off. She has turned that knot into a bow today.

I can't blame UJ for what happened on her first bus ride home from school. I waited for her at the bus stop, and waited, and waited. A bus stopped, but my daughter was not on it. Where was she? Which bus was she on? I called her school, and no one knew. Forty-five minutes passed and my six-year-old couldn't be traced. I imagined that her worst fear, now mine, had come true—that she blithely got off the bus who-knows-where in the city and was roaming the streets alone. In pure panic, I ran up and down a parallel bus route that goes through our neighborhood. I was wearing a black polyester shirt with tiny white flowers and worked myself up into a great sweat.

Then a miracle happened. UJ saw me. She was on the wrong bus, on another route that was forty minutes behind schedule, and she happened to catch a glimpse of me from outside the window. Now, this is a child with a reputation for being the dreamiest of space cadets. She's like a balloon that bobs above everything, casually oblivious, and she *saw* me—or, rather, my back—from afar. This kid, once distinguished by her reserve, shouted to the bus driver to let her off—*My mama's outside*—and he did.

Never before had my child been that alert or forceful in a new situation. Was it the novelty of riding the bus for the first time? The anxiety-as-excitement cognitive reappraisal trick I had suggested that morning? Was it chemosignals from other anxious kids who were taking the bus for the first time making her more with-it and vigilant? The right dose of cortisol? No matter. It was her first solo trip, and she soared.

Alas, *I* had crashed. I hadn't even seen her until she pulled my black polyester shirt from behind and shouted, "Mama! Why were you walking away?" When I saw her, I lunged and hugged her more tightly than ever, shaking, and my panic went straight to her core. She tensed up in bewilderment, then dissolved into tears. Suddenly, she felt responsible for getting on the wrong bus. She saw it as her performance failure—and mine, too, of course. "You were walking away! I saw your back!" she cried over and over again.

Just as panic can easily tip into excitement, so can excitement transmute to panic, and this is exactly what happened. Cortisol went from optimal to excessive; the butterflies in the stomach turned back into buzzards. She spent the rest of the afternoon in her room, under her triangle-motif comforter, ignoring my efforts to draw her out.

"I'll never take the bus again," she muttered from under the layers.

"Never?"

"Never in the universe."

My ultimate hope has been that if a kid learns to inure herself to the ups and downs of performance anxiety, she'll learn to be braver and take more risks. At this moment, it seemed she'd take fewer.

I tried the cognitive reappraisal tricks that I thought helped her violin performance. *Reframe it.* "That was so exciting!" I soothed. "I happened to be there, at the right place and the right time, and you happened to see me. You were amazing!"

She gave me a dead-fish-eyed look.

"It *was* exciting, wasn't it? Makes a good story with a good ending, right?"

Nothing.

So I resort to the old fallback: the fantastical. "Hey," I said. "If taking the bus from school is too stressful, what about taking a spaceship through outer space? NASA is looking for kid volunteers who'd be OK spending their lives going to Mars."

For all this talk of how the body can calm the panicked brain, so it seems can the idea of being weightless, disconnected, far away from an earthbound, flesh-bound reality.

A spaceship! I saw a little tremor of excitement under the comforter. "Yes," she said in an excited little-girl whisper. "Of course I'd do that!" When it comes to the ultimate risk for a human to take, to leave Mother Earth, there is "never never."

The next day UJ took the bus home again. I watched it approach at a snail's pace, yellow lights flashing. UJ was in the front seat behind the driver with her seatbelt tightly buckled. The bus pulled over slowly, the driver helped her unfasten the belt, and finally he opened the door to let her out. She stepped off and received my hug passively.

The ride was boring.

"Mama?" she said as we walked the four blocks home from the bus stop. I noticed that she was gripping the straps of her green backpack to avoid holding my hand.

"Next time, could I walk home alone?"

IV

Rebalance

———

OCTOBER

City Brain

Urban kids have unique brain wiring. Can the right words help prevent it from short-circuiting?

I F A SIX-YEAR-OLD with a mile-long gaze were walking alone on the city street, would strangers assist her, or would something unspeakable happen? I had asked myself that question last month when I thought my daughter got off the school bus at the wrong stop. Then it occurred to me that this scenario had already played out in a famous experiment staged by psychologists in the late 1970s. On the sidewalks of Manhattan, Philadelphia, and Boston, a frightened little kid cried, "I'm lost! Can you call my house?" You can imagine horns honking, towers looming, traffic, and choking fumes. Fourteen child actors—white, black, girls, boys—played the part of the lost child on different days. Some passersby swerved off the sidewalk to avoid the encounter with the child, even when the kid explicitly called to them, and some flat-out refused. "I'm lost too," one passerby snapped.

Of all the people the child appealed to for help, only about one-third stopped to offer any assistance. When the same experiment was done in smaller towns, 72 percent of the passersby helped. It's as Noël Coward predicted: "The higher the buildings, the lower the morals."

I loved the city more before I had kids. I came to New York for the culture, the diversity, the energy, the opportunities. Only in parenthood did I become so aware of the downside: the crowds, the cost, the noise, the fumes, and the competition over everything from obstetricians to kindergarten placement. Too many young people here seem bratty and entitled, or pushed and pressured, and everyone's in a self-possessed rush. Last week at the supermarket a woman slammed baby Ami's head with an oversized tote and didn't deign to stop and see what she hit.

You've got to wonder what the city does to the young brains for whom this is the native habitat. The answer is deeply relevant to more than half the world's parents, for we urbanites now outnumber the rest of the population. By 2050, nearly 70 percent of humans will live in cities. Many of us didn't grow up in a city but are raising city kids. The mental health stats are sobering. City kids are almost twice as likely to suffer from a psychotic episode as country kids (7.4 percent versus 4.4), and the difference isn't only due to socioeconomic factors. Meanwhile, adults living in the city have greater incidence of mood disorders (by almost 40 percent) and anxiety (by 21 percent) compared to those who live elsewhere. They're twice as likely to be schizophrenic.

I think I speak for most urban parents when I say we want better for our kids. We seek a brain-saving intervention that's easy, low-cost, effective, and doesn't require moving the kids to the suburbs, or even out of the apartment.

It just needs to move their minds.

Biology gives you a brain. Life turns it into a mind.
—Jeffrey Eugenides

Did you grow up in the city, the country, or the suburbs? If Andreas Meyer-Lindenberg, Florian Lederbogan, and their collaborators at the University of Heidelberg's Central Institute of Mental Health recruited you, that's the big question you'd have to answer. If you lived in the city, you'd tell them for how long and other details like your family income when you were little, your ethnicity, and other socioeconomic factors. The research team wanted to find out how much the city's stresses might affect the brains of relatively privileged middle-class white people versus their peers who grew up in other places. They wanted to make fair comparisons, so they were careful to make sure that there were no big differences in their subjects' mental health, mood, personality dimensions, or social support. Everyone grew up in a basically safe and comfortable-enough setting.

Then it was time to seriously stress those subjects out. A good way to do that, the team decided, was to make them take a computerized mental math test under time pressure. The test was designed to ask questions just beyond the subject's mental capacity, and the ticking clock intensified the agony. Then they added a special sadistic twist. In between series of questions, each test taker was made to feel that he or she couldn't measure up to the others. He or she would receive sharp feedback delivered through headphones. *We notice this seems hard for you. You're much slower than anyone else. You're in the bottom quarter. You're going to ruin the experiment. Try harder!* The test takers overheard the researchers talking among themselves, saying things such as *I can't believe he got that one wrong!* The point was to make the subject feel pushed, inadequate, and harshly judged.

As you might expect, the test was getting under the participants' skin: their hearts were beating faster, their blood pressure was higher, and they had higher circulating cortisol levels. And their minds? The research team also used fMRI to view brain activity during the experiment, and to see if there was any connection with the subject's childhood address. Could researchers tell which subjects had grown up in a city?

After the brain scan data were crunched, the researchers were so astounded by the differences that they ran the test twice, with more than one set of subjects, and then tested again. In urbanites, the amygdala—where fear, anxiety, and arousal are processed—was highly active during the test. City dwellers showed far more amygdala activity than those who lived in the burbs, who in turn showed more amygdala activity than those who lived in the country. And the larger the city in which a person lived, the more amygdala activity. This is particularly rattling for New Yorkers like me and my family, who live in a metropolis of roughly 8.5 million people.

This brings up the next question. Are city people (even relatively privileged ones) wired for stress in childhood, or do we just get that way after we move here?

Enter the ex-city kids, the other group in Meyer-Lindenberg and Lederbogen's experiment. They'd spent much or all of their early years in an urban area but as adults lived in the suburbs or country. Like the other subjects in the experiment, including urbanites who hadn't grown up in a city, they had a frustrating time with the mental math. They, too, were told that they weren't performing as well as the others and were treated with contempt.

Again, the neuroscience world was struck by what showed up in the brain scans. Ex-city kids—even if they had moved out to the hinterlands long ago—showed a unique pattern of brain activity when they thought they weren't measuring up. A region of their brain called the perigenual anterior cingulate cortex (pACC) was as active as a beehive. This same region was relatively quiet in all other groups, including the people who currently lived in a city but weren't born in one. The study concluded that the more years a person spent in the city as a kid, the more active the pACC was under stress. Unlike the amygdala, the pACC appears to be programmed in childhood and heavily influenced by childhood environment.

The pACC is involved in stress regulation and social processing: self-monitoring, watching one's own behavior, and storing emotional memories. Many neuroscientists think of the pACC as the brain's "social ladder," so it doesn't seem a stretch to imagine that when it's active, or overactive, as it was in people who had an urban upbringing, it's working hard to sort out one's place in the pecking order or to get a grip on what's going on in the social environment.

The brain scan images also picked up another potentially troubling difference among the ex-city kids. Normally, the pACC works closely with the amygdala to sort through social signals. Think of it as the "social sensitivity circuit." The pACC dials down an alarmed amygdala by sending it "braking" signals, thereby preventing the amygdala from reacting and triggering a negative emotion. Most subjects had a normal pACC-amygdala circuit, including those who currently live in the city. But people who'd grown up in the city, even after they'd moved away, had a thinner, weaker fiber connection between the pACC and amygdala. A weak link is associated with problems with emotional processing and is common among people at a genetic risk for mood disorders, including bipolar disorder and schizophrenia. It means that the pACC has less control over an overwrought amygdala, which helps to explain why a person might overreact to social stress.

But how can we be sure it was *social* stress that got to the former city kids, not performance stress? To find out, the team staged another experiment in which subjects had to take a difficult memory test, but this time they were spared the belittling put-downs and unflattering upward comparisons. Would the pACC in the former city kids still show signs of being overactive?

In short, no, it did not. Under normal performance pressure, the pACC in everyone, regardless of where they'd grown up, showed a normal level of activity, even if their amygdala was all abuzz. This supports the hunch that unusually strong *social* pressures of an urban childhood shape the pACC circuit. Because the pACC processes the perception of social status, city kids may have greater anxiety about not keeping up in some way—and it sticks for life. (A later study adds to the evidence, finding that psychosocial stressors raise cortisol levels in people who were raised in the city more than in those who grew up elsewhere, even if they currently live in a city. However, when city kids grew up and moved out, their brains showed less amygdala activity than current urbanites' did, suggesting that suburban or rural life offers some protection.)

For my daughters' sake, I worry about how the city might harm their social-sensitivity circuit. You can grow up anywhere and suffer from unflattering social comparisons and social pressures, of course. But perhaps one key difference in the city is that the comparisons are in one's face, all the time, often literally, due to the physical density and greater number of interpersonal encounters in their impression-able early years. The competition-cooperation ratio gets a little wonky. Who's smartest, richest, coolest, best dressed, best connected? Add to this a great deal of emphasis on socioeconomic status even among the very young, and you get a volatile mix of toxic exposures. A parent I know recalled her horror when her fifth grader said, with slit-eyed contempt, "We're taking JetBlue to Antigua? But I don't want to fly commercial!" (The researchers did not include inner-city subjects who grew up poor and nonwhite, but one can imagine the impact of more serious psychosocial stressors.)

The physical onslaughts of city life, including the density, noise, air pollution, and the scarcity of resources might also inflict wear-and-tear on a child's developing pACC-amygdala circuit. Imagine the honking and the catcalls; the pot smokers and the smoking tailpipes; the bobbing and weaving, the lack of green space and open skies, the homeless guy clutching a hot dog and aiming it like a gun at passersby (true story)—they all take an incremental toll on kids' psyches. The most direct walk home from UJ's school is a siren-filled stretch of avenue lined with monolithic high-rises. We pass a daycare center, a dry cleaner, a vegan takeout shop that looks and smells like a bank, several actual banks, a pharmacy, then, finally, a cancer clinic—all part of the same collection of cool, clean, subdued, mirror-tinted buildings. The corridor, I now realize, feels like a sinister analogy for life (and the donut shops are gone due to rising rents). UJ falls silent, plodding along, and even little Ami stares straight ahead in her carriage like one of those stunned blinkered horses in Central Park.

The famous psychologist Stanley Milgram once proposed that city life pushes the brain into "urban overload," which affects the way we process reality. Urban overload is a big reason, Milgram said, why so many city folk wouldn't even stop to help a lost kid. The poor amygdala is overstimulated, and the knee-jerk reaction is to block out stimuli.

One study showed that it only takes a momentary invasion of one's personal space—people standing too close—for the pACC-amygdala circuit to become stimulated. It's simply an evolved response to threat. Every rush hour on the subway, we're pressed up against other passengers so tightly that we can smell their incense or kielbasa sweat. Overload the circuit all the time with such stimuli and too little reprieve, and it becomes as worn out as the suspension on a yellow taxi.

Notwithstanding these stresses, I think it's extreme—and misguided—to presume that the city brain is a *weaker* brain. Many balanced and successful people grew up in a city, and still live there as adults. They're resilient and confident. I've wondered if there's an unsung upside of a prickly pACC: a superior awareness of social nuances. If you encounter hundreds of strangers every day, as my kids do—on the subway, at the bakery, on the streets, shouting *Hey, Princess, I love you! Hug me!*—you need the skills to size them up and tell who's trustworthy or kind or helpful—or not. Maybe, while you're at it, you also get better at evaluating complex social situations and scaling the social ladder. The jacked-up amygdala, meanwhile, may be at the heart of what my husband, a former city kid, calls "edge." An animal that grows up in an environment that's threatening or fiercely competitive may be savvier even if at times more insecure.

In the best of worlds, city kids would strike a Goldilocks balance: social sensitivity without runaway vulnerability. What determines where your city kid or mine falls on the continuum are the "mitigating factors": protection from poverty and racism; a sense of meritocracy; a safe and secure home; space and exercise; and a reduction in noise, pollution, and eyesores. Yet if I were asked to identify the bottom line, I'd bet on emotional resilience (a quality that the current research doesn't take well enough into account). It's all about a sense of personal control over one's fate.

When I look at emotional-resilience interventions that are easy to do in a New York moment, and that are well-researched, one stands out in all-caps: THE RIGHT STORY.

You may not control all the events that happen to you, but you can decide not to be reduced by them. —Maya Angelou

Once upon a time, right before Halloween, a hollowed-out red-haired man was sitting on our stoop. He was smoking a cigarette. Our family doesn't mind it when people take a break on our steps, but we're tired of sweeping up cigarette butts, and we hate the fumes that drift inside the building. "Excuse me," UJ said. "Please don't smoke on our steps." The man looked at the little girl with brown bangs and a tie-dyed shirt, and heaved a heavy sigh. "I'm sick," he told her. His face was mottled and his skin was slack. He was twining and untwining his bony fingers. UJ took a step back, and we walked up the steps quietly.

Later, the encounter struck a chord of anxiety in UJ. "What did he mean by 'sick'?" she asked. "Was I mean? Was he going to hurt us?"

The urban environment is full of stories, says Jan Golembiewski, the director of psychological design at Queensland University of Technology in Australia. In Golembiewski's view, we—our amygdalas—more often interpret what we encounter in the city as malevolent, even if we don't realize it. The wash of faces, the congestion and construction, the lurking doormen, the probing security cam, the sirens, the aggressive ads, the signs of out-of-reach affluence—they're all part of an urban narrative. In city life versus nature, he says, we're likelier "to identify stories that work against us, and they take a toll on our psyches." When we worry about wear-and-tear on the pACC-amygdala circuit, this is surely part of it.

Stories help children develop a theory of mind, the ability to understand others' actions and perspectives. They help kids learn compassion for others and for themselves. "Throughout evolution," Golembiewski writes, "stories have had the power to save us, because instinct is tied to narrative."

So, what if a kid could gain more control over those stories? What if she could make those stories work *for* her rather than against her? One way to protect the city brain, advises Golembiewski, is to essentially reframe, or replace, the city's aggressive barrage of messages with stronger personal narratives. The act of telling one's own story gives the urban amygdala what it so desperately needs: a reprieve. Finding descriptive words helps us to make sense of ourselves and the world.

Golembiewski has a name for this: narrative-enriched downtime. Little kids narrate effortlessly. Once upon a time, in our house, everything had a voice: the puppets and dolls, of course, but also the indignant eggs on the plate; the overeager pink hairbrush, Brusha, on which UJ drew an impish smiley face; and the greedy, narcissistic washcloth that shirked its butt-wiping duties. They often spoke on behalf of the preschooler herself. The kid controlled the message. But that power is used less with age, I realize with wistful regret. As UJ's awareness of the world expands, it has become more fact-oriented and less story-based. But it may be less personal and less comforting, too.

That's a loss, because the mental health benefits of expressive narratives (sometimes called anxious reappraisal) have gained credibility in neuroscience and psychology in recent years. This alone isn't news to me, and probably isn't to you, but the handful of studies on children or young teens is eye-opening because I had always thought of expressive narrative, especially when written, as an adult therapy.

Much of our understanding of how this brain hack works comes from the lab of James Pennebaker, a psychologist at the University of Texas at Austin whose experiments loosely follow these guidelines: Subjects are given a sheet of paper and a pen and are instructed to write, without any regard for spelling or grammar, a story about something that has happened to them. It might be a traumatic event or just something personal that they'd like to get out. They must write for fifteen to twenty minutes a day, for two to four days, about a stressful event in their lives.

The Pennebaker lab, and many others, shows that the act of translating feelings into words leads to superior emotional regulation. It's a step toward desensitizing oneself to the stress of whatever happened. It's an act of cognitive reappraisal, like when we reframe anxiety as excitement. Using language to reframe the confusing jumble of things they see or overhear or experience firsthand, kids create a version of reality that *they* control. They can tell the story of the homeless man with the hotdog or the story of the former best friend who became a hurtful gossip. They can write about losing the chess match, being rejected by the in-crowd, or feeling alienated at a swank birthday party. They can reframe painful situations in which they feel they weren't as smart or funny or rich or popular as others, and how they felt when they thought they fell short. Kids can put a word frame around the chaos of their lives. If they can curate it, they can master it.

I've often noticed that we are not able to look at what we have in front of us, unless it's inside a frame. —Abbas Kiarostami

It seems to me that the earlier in life a child learns cognitive reappraisal techniques, the better. The research shows that children as young as eight years old are capable of reframing their experience as a written story (and younger kids can try too, especially if the stories are told orally). A meta-analysis of twenty-one expressive-writing studies with ten- to eighteen-year-old subjects found that boys and girls who had a higher level of emotional problems at baseline showed better school performance and social adjustment after an expressive writing intervention compared to kids who already had good mental health, who often did not benefit.

But it seems safe to assume that, sooner or later, in any normal childhood—and maybe an urban one in particular—anxiety strikes. Then the goal for the child is to tame it before it outgrows his or her ability to control it. A few years ago, a team of psychologists led by Wendy Kliewer at Virginia Commonwealth University wanted to know if Pennebaker's expressive narrative intervention would help minority kids from low-income urban households who were exposed to high levels of community violence. The study included more than three hundred seventh graders who'd been frequently punched, chased, threatened—sometimes with a weapon—and seen the same happen to others at home or on the street. For twenty minutes, twice a week, for at least three weeks, some kids were randomly picked to write about their deepest, most painful thoughts about the worst things they'd seen or experienced, or anything else that was bothering them. (A control group wrote about nonemotional topics.) Later, teachers who were unaware of the study's hypothesis or what the kids wrote rated members of the expressive-writing group as acting less aggressive and emotionally volatile than the kids in the control group. Even two months after the last writing session, the expressive group remained less hostile and explosive than before the experiment, with the greatest improvement seen in the most aggressive kids (although no lasting benefit was seen at six months after the final writing session).

Because city kids' brains seem especially vulnerable to social stress, I perked up when I ran across an Italian study that looked at whether expressive writing offers any protection against bullying, social alienation, inferiority complexes, and other social stressors. The subjects here were all in seventh grade, and many felt they had been left out on purpose by other kids, were the victim of rumors, or were otherwise made to feel second-rate. By now I wasn't surprised to learn that the act of writing about their deepest, most troubling social conflicts (in four twenty-minute sessions over two weeks) helped these children cope better with their problems than those in the group told to write about trivial topics. Two months later, a postintervention assessment showed that the expressive writing group had developed more active coping strategies: positive reframing, problem solving, giving wider berth to toxic peers, and taking a more active stance against social stressors. Whether those strategies would eventually reduce anxiety and depression remains to be seen—they didn't in the span of this study. More long-term research is needed.

What has always seemed surprising (and, frankly, a little suspicious) to me in expressive writing studies is that there *are* long-term benefits. But in the dozens of studies using Pennebaker's method, you read about how subjects' blood pressure, heart rate, stress hormones, and sick days plummet for weeks and even months after they've assigned words to their feelings and stories to their words. No such link has been shown among the control groups that write about nonemotional topics. But how could a few short sessions of expressive writing about a troubling incident be therapeutic for so long? It sounds too good to be true.

There are several explanations. First, the writers (or storytellers) have off-loaded and processed the emotions, so they're less sensitized than when those feelings were bottled in. In communicating the troubling incident, they've shifted it in their head, so it's not the same as it was before the words were expressed, and never will be again. When it pops up in their minds again like the mole in whack-a-mole, as it will, they'll find that they have more than one way to contend with it. And now that they've relieved their working memory, which was chewing away on the problem in the background, they can devote those thought cycles to better things, which leads to thinking even less about the problem, and a virtuous cycle begins. Plus, since they've formally downloaded and reframed the story, this new version sticks better. (As Vonnegut said, "We are what we pretend to be, so we must be careful about what we pretend to be.")

Biohack: Rewriting (and Rewiring) the City Brain

To ascribe words to feelings is a biohack—the process "improves" one's brain circuitry. When kids label their emotions, a neural chain reaction is set in motion: first, the right ventrolateral prefrontal cortex kicks in, which helps them to transform their feelings into something to scrutinize or examine at a greater distance. The prefrontal cortex helps them realize that an experience may be stressful without losing themselves in their anxiety. This signal dials down the jumpy amygdala activity, even when, say, the pACC-amygdala circuitry is weak. As a result, the stress reaction is less knee-jerk.

There have been well over one hundred studies on the benefits of expressive writing, which has been found to benefit everything from working memory, to grades, to decreasing persistent negative thoughts and pretest math anxiety. (Note: It was not found to help with body image problems or to help kids without anxiety, and may have held back people who've recently been divorced or have PTSD, who may do better not to revisit painful stories.) Some studies have even linked expressive writing with higher grades in school. Pennebaker and other psychiatrists have established the following rules of thumb for writing about a source of anxiety, which I modified for kids:

- Set aside fifteen to twenty minutes for three or four days. This is the standard time for writing in the research studies, although one experiment found that as little as two minutes a day shows benefits. There are no set guidelines for children.

- A story must have a beginning, middle, and an end. No bullet points or idea fragments. This is one of those times when having a structure is important. In most studies the stories are based on personal experience, but for kids there's no rule against drawing on other people's stories too, or their reaction to other people's stories. Kids (and even adolescents) may need support to help them create a narrative or extract meaning from it.

- Some studies have found that writing longhand—which is better for younger kids than typing—is also more effective for emotion regulation (although typing is OK too). While most of the studies following Pennebaker's model involve writing, others have found that telling a story out loud is equally effective (and was the best approach for my first grader). The advantage of writing is that a kid can express a deep and personal thing privately without thinking about the reactions of parents or other adults.

- It's not English class. Tell the kid not to worry about punctuation, spelling, or grammar. Write continuously and repeat ideas if running short and there's still time on the clock.

- Use emotion words as much as possible (*happy, care, love, perplexed, embarrassed, unsure, awkward*). In several studies, the more people used positive emotion words in telling their story, the more their health improved, although even negative emotion words were associated with health improvements. Other research has found that when people are talking about their *happiest* times, they reap more benefits from talking about it, or replaying it, than writing about it.
- Use causal and insight-oriented words (*because, therefore, effect, understand, realize, know*). These are associated with the best outcomes.
- For younger kids, space out the sessions more than one day apart instead of consecutive days to allow time to process the feelings that have been stirred up. This may help the reframing effort.

Because children are the focus here, a special mention should be made for studies that found a benefit of expressive writing for kids who are anxious before taking tests. University of Chicago psychologists Gerardo Ramirez and Sian Beilock realized that when kids feel pressured to perform, their working memory is quickly depleted. With worry hogging so much mental bandwidth, it's hard to juggle numbers and concepts. In the study, the research duo had ninth graders take a high-stakes math exam under high and low performance pressure, and with or without a ten-minute Pennebaker-style writing exercise beforehand. Some of the students were asked to express their worries on paper. (*I'm afraid I'm going to make a mistake. I'm nervous about what's going to happen if I fail.*) Students most prone to worry benefited the most from the exercise, achieving math scores that were significantly higher than those of their peers who hadn't downloaded their worries beforehand (an average grade around 90 percent versus 82 percent).

Still skeptical? Even after more than one hundred studies have been published on the effectiveness of expressive writing in various situations—most of which have found anywhere from a slight to strong benefit—we (OK, I) want further proof. This is the age of the quantified self, and psychologists (not to mention parents) are eager to see evidence in the form of measurable changes in the brain.

So, UCLA's Social Cognitive Neuroscience Lab staged an experiment in the school's fMRI brain-mapping room. First, they flashed photographs of angry and threatening faces in the faces of volunteers. Everyone's amygdala showed strong activity, as expected. Then, they asked the subjects to attach expressive words to the images: *angry, fearful, scornful,* and so on. Almost instantly, the brain activity changed. Words—expressive, emotive words!—deactivated the amygdala. At the same instant, a region of the brain involved in emotion regulation, the right ventrolateral prefrontal cortex, showed signs of activity. These brain changes did not occur when the subjects linked any other types of words, like names, with the disturbing faces.

It's a powerful idea, that the simple act of assigning emotive words to feelings protects the amygdala. This is relevant to younger kids, even those of preschool age, who might not be up to the task of constructing a story. When Ami throws her food on the floor, I label the emotion. *Frustrated! Ami is frustrated!* (It's a phrase she now owns and gleefully shouts even as she's breaking things.) When she sabotages UJ's art project I say, *Jealous! Ami is jealous because Ami wants to paint too.* But the single-word label acts as a shorthand with UJ, too, when there's no time or inclination for the whole-hog narrative reframing exercise.

One day after school I force an end to an impromptu playdate, and UJ cries out in anger and agony. One of the girls she had been playing with snorts and says, in what I think to be a pejorative tone, "It's OK, really, you'll be OK, you'll get to see us tomorrow." UJ still has crying jags as we walk away, so I ask her to assign some words to the incident to describe how she feels:

"Embarrassed. Awkward. Frustrated. Annoyed," she says, sniffling. "And deforested."

"Deforested?"

"Yes, Mama, it's a metaphor." And she laughs; something has shifted.

Speaking of social life, I want to know if there is any evidence that expressive writing might help city kids' touchy social-status sensor, the pACC. So, I look for a brain imaging study and find one that took place at the University of Ulm, in Germany. In this setup, volunteers were shown cards—for instance, a person sitting alone on a bench—accompanied by versions of the story that described what was going on in an either abstract or emotional way. Volunteers read the story cards, and when there was emotional content ("she expresses total desperation sitting on this bench"), their scans revealed activation in the amygdala and pACC, among other regions. Afterward, the subjects were instructed to write what they remembered about the story in their own words.

The upshot was that when people used abstract or merely descriptive words, the pACC-amygdala circuit stayed on. But when they chose to use emotional words to recall the stories (*helpless, terrified, forlorn, uncertain, sorrowful, safe*), both the pACC and amygdala *deactivated*. This is potentially good news to those worried about their city kid developing a weak pACC-amygdala circuit. It suggests that when children (and adults) use high-emotion words to express troubling emotions, there's less wear and tear on the pACC and amygdala. It gives that circuit a much-needed break for mental health.

As always, I make a plea for further research. On my wish list is a study that would test whether expressive language helps in a moment of social anxiety—say, when a child or teenager feels belittled, jealous, like an imposter, or that she's falling short in some way. The theory is that constant stress on a city kid's pACC-amygdala circuit wears it out, which only furthers social anxiety and the stress of always measuring up. Over time, I wonder, could the use of expressive language help strengthen and preserve the circuit?

**There is no calamity which right words will not begin to redress.
—Ralph Waldo Emerson**

When UJ's encounter with the sick red-haired guy on our city stoop continued to haunt her even a day later, she redressed. Her story, constructed while walking home from school, was a twist on Pennebaker's approach: emotive and reflective but also reinventive. It was as much a story about the sick man in the city as it was about her:

> On Halloween, many years ago, in a little cottage on a mountain top, a mama rocked her redheaded baby. There were blazes of red and yellow and orange leaves everywhere. When the boy was six, his cottage burned down, his world went up in flames, and the mama was gone. The boy moved to the city, where he began to smoke to forget his worries, but cigarettes made him sick. Then, one day, he sat on my stoop and met me on my way home. I was scared of him at first. I was a little disgusted. My mama didn't see him as well as I did, but he was really sick, and I could see that, and my heart swelled. So he moved in, and now he sleeps in our spare bed. I am helping him get healthy again with miso soup, and I won't let him smoke anymore.

Afterward, she let out a moan of dismay. "I wish we had his phone number so we could find him!" (May no heartless cad ever take advantage of her.)

Storytelling helps us to connect the city with our interior world. Who on the train looks like they're having a bad day? What happened? Why is that man homeless? How did that violinist on the corner get so good? Sometimes the subject is the kid herself. Sometimes the story is just one word. *Overwhelmed.*

When there's flow (there isn't always, and I've learned it can't be forced), "narrative enrichment" is magical. My daughter is less moody. She holds my hand when we walk. All is cool on the social-stress circuit. The golden autumn light shines down in these moments, and even with all the shouts and sirens and smog, it feels like the city is a land of happily ever after. The type of place where, even if a kid gets lost, she'd find her way back home.

NOVEMBER

Rage Against the Dying of the Light

_____

Change the lightbulb, change the thinker?

A S THE OIL of Olay commercial put it, "I don't intend to grow old gracefully. I intend to fight it every step of the way." That's how I feel about the fading sunlight, the year's visible wind down. It started in unnoticeable increments, three minutes a day since late September. Then, in the wee hours of the first Sunday of this month, daylight saving time officially ended, and we were robbed of an entire hour of afternoon light. Now darkness falls devastatingly early—before five o'clock—and the night will arrive earlier and earlier until the winter solstice, December 21, the shortest day in the year.

It's only UJ's seventh trip around the sun, but I don't want to shield her from life's harsh realities. She's old enough now to understand what we're up against. One evening this month, I hold up my fist to represent the sun, and draw her attention to the 23.5-degree tilt of her globe. "Look, look what happens! The sun is *here* and we live *here*, in the United States, in the Northern Hemisphere. See how we're tilted away from the sun right now? That means we get fewer hours of daylight at this time of year. See how the Southern Hemisphere, South Africa and Argentina and Australia, is tilted toward the sun now? See how when it's spring here, it's fall there? And when it will be summer there, it will be winter here? Soon, too soon."

"Mama. Move to Australia."

But no, we've stayed and battled the dark forces with every tool in our arsenal: twenty recessed ceiling lights, two chandeliers, a table lamp, and three floor lamps. Then, as pièce de résistance, three immense hanging globe lights outfitted with near-daylight-strength ultracompact fluorescent bulbs. Inside, we live in eternal summer.

It's no different at school. Thanks to ultrabright compact fluorescents and LEDs, the average classroom is brighter than ever. And not just bright but illuminated with the sort of energizing short wavelength cold blue light that penetrates deeper into the eye than light of other wavelengths.

But at what sacrifice? To paraphrase Rachel Carson, humans are part of nature, and to go to war against nature is, inevitably, to go to war against ourselves. This fall, the kids have had little exposure to actual sunlight. The availability of electricity and cheap, intense bulbs has made us creatures of the brightest light without any connection to the spinning planet we live on or the sun that makes life possible.

Children might not realize it, but the color, intensity, and quantity of daily illumination influences their mood and performance. Spending all their waking hours under bright fluorescent light may put them in a very different mindset from, say, six hours of indoor light and seven hours of (varying) outdoor light, much less living in more darkness this time of year, the way our ancestors did before electricity. What do our children stand to lose, or to gain, by spending so much of their childhood like broiler chicks under the henhouse lamps? Is there any upside to reclaiming the darkness? If you change the lightbulb, do you change the thinker?

A rock pile ceases to be a rock pile the moment a single man contemplates it, bearing within him the image of a cathedral.
—Antoine de Saint-Exupéry

Over the past few years, several researchers have looked more closely at how the color temperature of light affects how people think and act. Color temperature isn't a measure of a lightbulb's heat but its hue, measured in degrees kelvin (K). As counterintuitive as it sounds, the "cooler" the hue, the higher the color temperature. Most standard indoor white light runs within the range of 2,700 K (warm, yellow-ish) to 5,000 K (cold blue). The eight compact fluorescent bulbs over my family's kitchen area emit 2,700 K each. To give you an idea of the scope, candlelight is 1,500 K, the blue sky is 9,000 to 12,000 K, and the blue inner core of a flame is about 6,000 K—which, like your computer or TV screen, can keep you up later in the night. Institutional lighting, too, runs toward the cooler, bluer side of the spectrum. This means that kids spend hours of their school day, a large chunk of childhood, awash in artificial high-K blue light.

What does all that light do to children's ability to think? That was my first question, and I found some answers in a joint study by Cornell, the University of Irvine, and the software giant Microsoft. The research team staged an experiment in which volunteers (all adults, alas) were exposed to an extra twenty-minute dose of high-intensity 5,000 K light at their desks on certain days. Then, for each day of the ten-day study, the volunteers took two standardized psychological tests to assess different aspects of creativity.

The first test, known as the Compound Remote Associates Test, measured convergent thinking, which requires focus to get to the one right answer. The subjects needed to find the matching term that combines with three words in a set. Here's one to try on a kid: What word unites *cream/skate/water*? If the child answers *ice*, he's thinking convergently. A nerdy kid might recognize and possibly enjoy this type of problem. (UJ did.) Convergent thinking is a form of creativity, but it's limited because there's only one correct answer to a problem.

Given the surge of energy and focus we feel under a blue sky, or when walking into a big-box fluorescent-lit store late at night, it may come as no surprise that the study showed that bright, cold light leads to better convergent thinking. Test takers scored nearly 25 percent better on the Compound Remote Associates Test on extra-blue-light days than on control days when there was no extra blue light, and they had more eureka moments. (What links *aid/rubber/wagon*? Aha! *Band!*) Convergent thinking has also been found to be helpful for arithmetic, multitasking, decision making, and acing multiple-choice questions.

When researchers look at brain scans of people exposed to bright light, they see greater activation in regions of the prefrontal cortex involved in arousal and attention. Some studies (although not all) find that working memory improves significantly. Working memory is a big part of convergent thinking, because you need to draw on long-term memory, and then mentally manipulate that information to get to the one right answer. Some researchers also credit a hormonal response to blue light driven by melanopsin, the protein in retinal cells that detects that wavelength. Melanopsin indirectly triggers a neurotransmitter, norepinephrine, which makes us more alert and aware. Norepinephrine is also a working memory enhancer.

For many parents and educators, the evidence that blue light helps kids do better on intense working memory–based activities is a real bright spot, especially since the research is fairly robust. The brighter and bluer, the better, or so it seems. When Korean fourth graders took timed math tests under cold daylight-strength LED lights (6,500 K), they scored better than under 3,500 K lights, the usual classroom fluorescents. Similarly, when Dutch scientists ratcheted up the blue experimental lighting to the same 6,500 K, students outperformed their peers who took the same high-concentration tests in regular school lighting of 4,000 K.

Let's see what else blue light can improve, as shown in the scientific literature. Remote word association: check. Multiple choice: check. Concentration: check. Math: check. Problem solving: check. Faster decision making and response time: check.

How about reading fluency? This one's interesting because a lot of subtle cognitive horsepower goes into reading a text automatically and accurately. The less a child stumbles over syllables or pauses to decode a word or parse a sentence, the more bandwidth she can devote to comprehending the text. In the experiment, which extended over the school year, four classes of third graders took reading lessons in which they had fluency instruction. Two classrooms used "focus" lights: brilliant white 6,000 K bulbs (during the instruction only, not the rest of the day), while the other two classrooms used the regular school lighting of 3,500 K. Later in the year, the experimenters came in to have the kids read graded passages aloud and calculated the numbers of words read correctly.

While all tests were conducted under regular classroom lighting, the difference between the two study groups was striking. The kids who had taken reading lessons under the bright focus lights showed a 36 percent increase in performance over the year, while the group with the normal 3,500 K lights showed only a 17 percent improvement. What exactly were they better at? Recognizing words and matching them to the right expression, intonation, and timing, which shows that they understood the text and the implied tone. To do this, cognitive and linguistic skills need to work smoothly and in concert. Again, this is where convergent thinking shines.

However, when you cast more light on people's performance under bright blue lights, you'll find shades of gray. Some studies find that the blue-light benefit lasts at least forty minutes after exposure and that performance is best in that cooldown spell after the bright-light episode, not *during* it. For many people, bright light in the morning was more effective than in the afternoon. There's also new evidence that the blue-light boost is bigger when a person is already alert and the task isn't too difficult, because it can nudge him or her to that sweet spot of arousal. If the task is too challenging and complex, blue light might backfire and push a thinker into a state of overarousal. (Remember the Yerkes-Dodson Law? You want to be in the arousal sweet spot: not too much and not too little.) Then, the strategy doesn't seem so bright.

To cease to think creatively is but little different from ceasing to live. —Benjamin Franklin (attributed)

For every yang, there's a yin. If convergent thought is on one side of the spectrum, the opposite is *divergent* thought, and there's reason to believe that blue light eclipses it. Divergent thinking is spontaneous, free-flowing, freewheeling, playful, and nonlinear. We want our kids to wear their divergent thinking caps when they need to solve a problem and the solution isn't clear-cut or when more than one solution is right. Divergent thinking leads to the eureka moment when UJ spins a poem out of air, or when Ami, desirous of a bagel on the counter and denied a stepstool, pulls out the drawers and makes them into steps.

The second creativity test in the blue-light study was the Unusual Uses Task (the same test used in the daydream study we explored in May). This is a divergent thinking test, and subjects had to answer questions such as *How many uses can you come up with for a shoe?*

They had four minutes to brainstorm ideas, which were judged not by quantity but by novelty. A convergent thinker would think up variants on foot protection—running, mountain climbing, ballet, and so on; after all, those are logical and relevant uses for a shoe. But a divergent thinker would imagine scores of unexpected, possibly crazy uses—say, a safe place to hide money, raw material for a playground surface, a source of foot odor to make tick repellant.

When it came to thinking up unexpected uses for a shoe and other common objects, the thinkers' thoughts seemed to depend a great deal on the lighting. The same twenty minutes of blue light that helped them in the convergent thinking test appeared to hobble them when it came to thinking up divergent ideas. On the days with the extra blue light, people thought of fewer novel and creative solutions for objects than they did on control days when there was no extra blue light. This triggered a serious question: Could blue light harm blue-sky thinking?

Try the Unusual Uses Task with your kid at home, under the blue light of midday or a bright fluorescent versus the glow of the night-light. *How many uses can you think of for a paperclip?* (A mini trombone? A headphone detangler? A cockroach pin?) Or try a variant such as *How many uses can you think of that combine a brick and a safety pin?* The more original and elaborate the idea, the higher the score. Does the child think more creatively in bright light versus dim? Or try another divergent thinking test, the Consequences test, developed by the Aptitudes Research Project at the University of Southern California. Ask questions such as *What would happen if everyone were immortal? What would happen if we had no teachers?* Does the child come up with richer, more unusual responses in the semidarkness? My daughter does.

Building on these findings, Anna Steidle and Lioba Werth, researchers at German universities, were curious if lighting affected the imagination—specifically, the ability to envision other worlds. They gathered students in their late teens and twenties and assigned them to rooms with normal, bright, or "dim" lighting. (The dim lighting was half the intensity of normal room lighting. *The Manual for Sacred Buildings* suggests this lighting level for a temple or church nave.)

The participants received a sheet of blank paper and instructions that read, "Imagine going to another galaxy and visiting another planet very different from Earth." Then they had seven minutes to draw the aliens they imagined they'd encounter. The judges scored the pictures based on creativity. How atypical were the aliens' bodies? What did the artists do about sensory organs? How unexpected was the placement of body parts? The odder they were, the higher the score.

As it turned out, the best "lightbulb moments" happened when the room was no darker than the average parking lot at night. In dim lighting the artists' alien renderings became notably more imaginative and atypical than in the normal and bright settings. While bright light promotes focus and vigilance, dim light appears to make a kid feel more relaxed, calmer, freer, and more likely to lower his or her guard. Like greenery and nature immersion, dim light appears to facilitate a default mode state—daydreamy, associative—while bright light increases focused, directed attention. The brighter the room light, the more the aliens resembled humdrum Earth creatures, albeit more detailed than the ones drawn in dimmer light. Steidle and Werth snuck in a logical reasoning test too, which the participants took right before they drew their aliens. Sure enough, the bright-room and the normal-room groups outperformed the dim-room group in these questions, which required focused attention.

The average kindergartener scores at genius level on divergent thinking tests. Ask five-year-olds what to do with dandelion fluff, and they'll tell you it's "Oof food" or angel bait or seeds for a wishing stalk. Five years later, at age ten or so, those same kids' scores drop by 50 percent. They struggle to come up with novel ideas. By the time they're in their midteens, their divergent thinking scores drop further, and only 10 percent score as geniuses. While convergent thinking is essential when taking standardized tests, divergent thinking is considered the number-one leadership competency of the future and is crucial for innovation. Creativity scores are declining among kids, and the overemphasis on convergent thinking in school is a threat to progress on a nationwide or even global level.

For facts, we have computers; for creative problem solving, we need flexible minds.

This is not to diminish convergent thinking. I'm just saying that it should share its pedestal in the educational spotlight. It should also be said that both divergent and convergent thought are necessary for creativity. While divergent thinking yields novel and possibly impossible, outlandish ideas, convergent thinking helps thinkers to pare those ideas down, give them structure, and make them useful. The most ingenious minds can be both spotlight and diffuser. Any parent, and certainly any educator, can see the value in striking the right balance.

To that end, most of us, I think, don't seriously consider the effect that the lighting spectrum has on the thinking spectrum. How many schools have considered that attention fatigue, so common among young students, may have at least something to do with light overstimulation?

Given that the mind uses light as a cue to be either vigilant and focused or free-ranging and undirected, why not experiment to get it right? Mix it up. Aim for periods of focused attention under bright daylight-mimicking lights. Keep those blue compact fluorescents and LED lights on during arithmetic, when absorbing facts, taking tests, and rebounding from the postlunch energy dip. Shift to dimmer, diffused lighting for creative thinking, problem solving when there's more than one solution, and when brainstorming together.

Problem is, it's easier to turn on the bright lights than to turn them off. Almost everyone's a blue-light addict.

Creativity—like human life itself—begins in darkness.
—Julia Cameron

It wasn't always so. At dinnertime, UJ slurps her chickpea soup with barley ("Swallow first, sweetie") and talks about a group presentation she is to give at school. Her class is learning about Native Americans, the Lenape, who lived in Manhattan and other parts of the Northeast before the Dutch arrived. In summer, she says, the Lenape would fish; in spring, they'd plant and hunt; and in the fall, they'd harvest corn, squash, and beans, hunt, and prepare for the winter. In winter, they'd bury food and sit in their wigwams.

"So what's your favorite season?" I ask, ever eager to talk about her day.

"Winter, definitely," UJ says seriously, slurping.

"Winter!" Ami repeats, grinning hard. Ami now has a disconcerting habit of repeating words we say and then laughing her head off. "*Winter! Winter!*"

"Why not summer?" I ask thoughtfully. To me, the Lenape winter sounds either boring or brutal.

"But," says UJ, "winter is the season for stories!"

My daughter has a sentimentalized snow-globe view of Lenape life. Night came on early, she explains, and the Lenape would retreat to their wigwams. There, storytellers would tell tales to the firelit audience: great ones about people who were punished for their greed or pride, or warnings about needless wars; or about the origins of things; or about the magical people of the woods who'd punish those who disrespected nature. The Lenape, who possibly lived on the very same plot of land we live on now, were cocooned in a dreamy membrane at this time of year. They told stories, went to sleep early, and dreamed.

Hearing this, it occurs to me that our enthusiasm for artificial lighting has nudged us far in the other direction. In the summer we stay up later and later naturally, but winter is a dreamier and more contemplative time. Ever since I've turned on the brightest lights to counter the dark and cold, UJ and Ami have suffered from evening mania. (Well, the parents have suffered; the kids love it.) The children vibrate through dinner and get increasingly wound-up afterward, streaking around and refusing to settle down. It's been weeks since UJ has been in the mood for the end-of-the-day reflection. Our bedtime storytelling sessions are shorter and brusquer. There's no evening enlightenment, just *light*. And, increasingly, a dark cloud over my head as I frantically spray magnesium onto the children's feet, rubbing harshly as I implore them to calm down and go to sleep.

The magnesium helps. But for better and for worse, they have not gone gentle into that good night.

That's because we live in melatonin-deprived times. If the hormone were a hero in a movie or a book, it'd be slow, heavy, and fuzzy. Melatonin is the underdog that carries us to the nether realms of sleep. It rises in the dark only. Its kryptonite is blue light, which is spreading everywhere on the planet as compact fluorescent and LED technology becomes cheaper and brighter. The blue light is destroying the planet's melatonin supply.

If we "rewilded" or went au naturel and turned the lights off from five o'clock at this time of year, the retinal cells in our eyeballs would detect the dimming sunlight. It'd pass on the news, via the optic nerve, to the blue-light-detecting suprachiasmatic nucleus (SCN) in the hypothalamus. The SCN, which controls circadian rhythms of night and day, would send signals to the pineal gland to secrete melatonin. The hormone would signal our neurons to slow down their electrical rhythms. As melatonin rises, our bodies shift down and eventually ease into sleep. We'd be down before our current dinnertime.

Would we value melatonin more if we knew that it reduces the ravages of the day: oxidative stress and inflammation? The hormone slows down cell division, which might help to explain why adults with low melatonin levels at night are likelier to have breast and prostate

cancers. The hormone keeps sex hormones in check, regulates the ova-
ries, and prevents eggs from maturing too quickly. In other mammals,
melatonin levels are relatively high in the winter, suppressing fertility.

Melatonin also influences the timing of puberty: girls' breast buds
and periods and boys' voice changes and testicular growth. There's a
link—terrifying, controversial, and largely unexplored—between early
puberty and low melatonin. The elementary-school-aged girls who
wear bras and use sanitary napkins have lower-than-average melatonin
levels, whereas girls with delayed puberty have higher-than-average
levels, and girls with normal pubertal development are somewhere in
the middle. (A curious link also exists between physical activity and
melatonin: the less exercise, the lower the hormone.)

Several studies also support the idea that lights at night interfere
with the sleep hormone enough to significantly mess with developmental controls. Streetlight glow, it seems, could explain why city birds
(pigeons, ravens, crows) have faster biological clocks than country
birds. They reach sexual maturity and lay eggs sooner. I don't wish
for my girls to be early birds at the dawn of adolescence.

Low melatonin only correlates with early signs of puberty, but
the stakes are high. While puberty accelerates brain development and
efficiency, it also means the end of the flexible, spongelike child brain
that absorbs new information and languages easily. As parents and
educators, we tend to focus on psychosocial difficulties of precocious
puberty, but there's also an enormous loss when a child's brain loses
its flexibility too early. Music, language, even creative problem solving
may become harder in some ways.

I've come to see melatonin as a necessary break. If light hurries us
up, melatonin slows us down. It may slow down puberty, slow down
cell division, slow down reaction time. It moves the mind toward
dreamtime, the absence of time.

I will love the light for it shows me the way; yet I will love the darkness because it shows me the stars. —Og Mandino

Without quality sleep, everything we care about falls apart: resilience, sociability, competence, character, connection, and self-control. (The American Academy of Pediatrics suggests eleven to fourteen hours for toddlers; ten to thirteen for three- to five-year-olds; nine to twelve for six- to twelve-year-olds; eight to ten for teenagers.) Adolescents have their melatonin peak two to three hours later than children and adults, which is one reason why they have trouble waking up in the morning. (This biological fact is driving a movement for later high school start times.)

We all know that blue-light wavelengths suppress melatonin, which in turn delays sleep. So, if we avoid blue screens or gas-station lighting at night, the kids are all right? Alas, it turns out that the pineal gland, where melatonin is produced, responds to the *intensity* of light that meets the eye, as well as the color temperature. What I didn't realize is that a light need not be a cool blue LED or a fluorescent to suppress melatonin; it can be white or yellow light, both of which have some energizing blue frequencies. Any light can suppress melatonin if it is intense enough to the retina.

The intensity of light is measured in lux. A lux meter, a standard tool in a photographer's camera bag, can be had for less than twenty dollars, so I buy one and measure the lux in every room of our house. My kitchen area, with bulbs at 2,700 K color temperature, clocks in at about 400 to 500 lux. The average home is about 300 lux, which is about the same intensity as twilight, and the average classroom is about 400 to 500 lux. As a point of comparison, the bright beach at midday can be 12,000 lux and higher, and midday sun near the equator is about 80,000 lux. A candle sheds a modest 3 lux.

My family normally hangs out in the kitchen area until bedtime. Two hours under my 500-lux lights, I learn from a Harvard study, can suppress a melatonin surge almost as effectively as one hour of light at 1,000 lux, which is the intensity you'd experience in an operating theater or outside on an overcast day.

What's cruel is that kids are doubly affected, because the same amount of light that delays an adult's melatonin rise delays theirs twice as long. Look into your child's big, crystalline eyes, and you'll see why. Children's pupils dilate at least 1.5 times wider than do adults' in all types of light. As a result, more light hits the retina, especially the stimulating blue-light wavelengths. The more light that hits the retina, the lower the melatonin.

In a Japanese study, 580 lux of light at night (not much more than what my daughters get at the dinner table) shut down children's melatonin rise by almost 90 percent in the hour or two before bed, compared to only 45 percent suppression in adults. Even in the kids' bedrooms, where the light intensity was an economical 145 lux in the hour before shuteye, melatonin was suppressed by 50 percent—twice as much as in adults—compared to 3 lux light. Such sensitivity doesn't end in puberty. In fact, a study found that early adolescents (nine- to fourteen-and-a-half-year-olds) are particularly sensitive to light. No matter the amount of lux—whether 50 or 500—light suppresses their melatonin levels significantly more than in older high schoolers.

Now I'm enlightened.

Biohack: Illuminating Thoughts

Light is one of the most powerful ways to hack a kid's mental (and physical) state. Maximize it for convergent thinking, and honor and optimize the dark for divergent thinking, quality rest, health, and resilience. Consider buying a lux meter, which costs as little as ten to fifteen dollars, to measure light intensity in your home. As the eponymous Lord Kelvin (after whom color temperature measurement was named) said, "If you can't measure it, you can't improve it." Here's what we do at night:

- Reduce exposure to all sources of short blue wavelengths at night because they suppress melatonin and disrupt sleep cycles. These include the usual suspects: computers, cell phones, and video-game screens. But most white light, including compact fluorescents, also includes energizing blue frequencies that suppress melatonin. Avoid curlicue compact fluorescents in favor of warmer energy-saving LED bulbs. At a minimum, wear orange-tinted, blue-light-blocking goggles or use software such as f.lux to "warm up" screens and avoid exposure to blue light at night.

- Gradually dim the lights in the two to three hours before bedtime. If you have dimmer switches, use them. If not, turn off the bright lights one by one. For our eight o'clock bedtime, this means turning off more lights every hour after six o'clock. In our home, by seven, our retinas are taking in only 50 to 100 lux (2,700 K). Use blackout shades to cut ambient glow, especially from the new high-powered fluorescent streetlights, which disrupt melatonin even from afar.

- For a radical reset of circadian cycles, take your children camping for four to five nights without any artificial lights. If that's not possible, keep the lights off after sunset and use a timer to raise the shades at dawn or use an artificial dawn-simulating light. The natural cycles of day and night sync even those with an "evening-oriented" chronotype with the earth's rhythms. There are fewer human night owls in the wild.

- If a child needs a night-light, use amber lights and filters to reduce the light to 5 lux or lower, the level of light intensity that will not affect working memory or sleep quality. We use an orange night-light and taped orange cellophane (from a bag) over the bedside clock. Light can suppress melatonin even through the eyelids.

In the first weeks after the clocks were set back this month, the mornings were a little brighter than before. But the light recedes a little each day, and by the end of the month, we rise in the dark once again. Well, *rise* may be overstating it. Some mornings UJ is awake enough to be snappish, especially when I'm trying to brush her hair, but then she shuts down during the commute. She arrives at school slightly stunned, blinking like a newborn. So this is what we'll do in the mornings until the spring equinox:

- While evening is the time to fuel melatonin, morning is the time to snuff it out with pure blue light. An optimal time for blue-light ex-posure is a half hour after waking. We're time crunched, so I bought an inexpensive blue light of 10,000 lux intensity and installed it near UJ's seat at the table so that she may eat her eggs in a futur-istic blue glow. Biologically speaking, the blue light immediately suppresses melatonin and triggers the morning spike in cortisol. When we think of cortisol, we think stress. But in the right doses, the hormone is also an energizing, nervous-system activator.

- When using an energizing blue light, try to position it from above. The most sensitive light receptors are in the lower area of the retina. (Although the companies that make the lights say they are safe for eyes, children are especially sensitive to UV light—one reason why their melatonin levels are more easily suppressed than in adults. As a precaution, don't position a bright light directly in a child's eyes.)

And during the day, try the following:

- Use daylight-strength (7,500 K, 500 lux or more) LED or compact fluorescent bulbs for attention, focus, and concentration. Alternate with dimmer, warmer light (50 to 100 lux) to encourage divergent thinking and to avoid mental fatigue. Use this light when your child is brainstorming or working on a creative project, and in that twilight stream-of-consciousness state before bed.
- If your child is working on a task that demands high-performance convergent thinking or great focus—math, word problems, fact finding, tests—consider exposing him or her to at least twenty minutes of cold blue daylight-strength light before he or she begins. Blue light has been found to arouse the brain for at least forty minutes after exposure.
- Aim for at least an hour of natural daylight every day for normal growth of the lens and retina. An Ohio State University study found that kids who spent at least two hours a day outdoors were four times less likely to be nearsighted than those who spent less than one hour. Nearsightedness is caused by elongation of the distance between the retina and lens. Exposure to natural light of multiple wavelengths stimulates retinal dopamine, which slows down this growth. Artificial light disrupts the retinal dopamine cycle. Vitamin D from sun exposure supports the muscles that tense around the lens of the eye, which keeps the parts in proper position even as a child grows rapidly.

Lights conquered darkness and all that lurked therein,
real or imagined. —Mark Bouman

The plan is to take back the night, light by light and lux by lux. It's called graduated bedtime, an incremental weakening of the houselights as the evening progresses. We're making our own artificial sunset.

Our home experiment is backed by research that shows that you can accelerate the onset of melatonin rise if you remember to dim the lights before bedtime. In one study, subjects who were exposed to just 3 lux at night, the equivalent of a night-light, had a melatonin onset an hour earlier than those who had been in a 65-lux room. Although the 3-lux group went to sleep only fifteen minutes earlier than usual, their reaction times the following morning were faster because they had been asleep during their restorative melatonin peak, and there had been no hiccup in their circadian timing.

It's not that kids *can't* sleep without a big melatonin rise. Fatigue or habit can put them down. But melatonin-light sleep is not necessarily the same quality rest as melatonin-heavy sleep. In lab experiments, when subjects must stay awake and miss the middle-of-the-night peak melatonin mark, their performance on cognitive tests is impaired the next day even if they sleep in.

Outside, when the sun sets relatively early, the early melatonin rise is even more profound. In a small experiment led by University of Colorado Boulder psychologists, volunteers camped in the mountains for a week without any artificial light, not even a flashlight. It was summer, and the campers would go to sleep naturally with the sun and wake up with it. The upshot is that *everyone*, morning larks and night owls alike, went to sleep earlier and slept longer. The researchers concluded that night owls (like me and both of my children) would find it hard to stay up without the electric lights that allow us to stray from the norm.

Going by one theory, evening-oriented types (10 to 15 percent of the population) evolved around the same time as the invention of fire four hundred thousand years ago. This subset of the population had eyes that were more sensitive than others to the blue light in the core of the fire, so their melatonin was suppressed more easily. (Are night owls that way because their retinas are more sensitive to light? Another study for the wish list.) The wee-hour vigilance may have been a good thing in a world in which predators or enemies struck at night. But it isn't for children who must be at school by eight o'clock—so, for a global reset, take them camping for a few nights or just turn off the lights at sunset. That should sync them to the early bird world.

In autumns past, especially before the blue-blasting lights, melatonin would kick in around six o'clock in the evening. I'm not willing to put the kids to sleep at that time. There are simply too many hours of darkness, and turning in that early would lead to biphasic sleep. The entire family would wake in the middle of the night for an hour or two to ponder and play, as they did in pre-electrified Europe, and then go back to sleep until morning. That schedule surely has its charms. But no. Here's the more practical version we do at home:

- By 5:30 it's dark outside. Inside, it's full-blaze. My lux meter registers about 500 lux for the combination of room lighting: the three 2,400 K spheres over the table, the recessed lights in the ceiling, and the compact-fluorescent bulbs in the floor lamps. It's OK; we still have two and a half hours to go before our target bedtime.
- By 6:00, I turn off the daylight-power globe lights above the kitchen table as well as the floor lamps, dimming the room down to 300 lux.
- By 6:30, I switch off the warm recessed LED ceiling lights in the room. My meter registers the light intensity at about 200 lux.
- By 7:00, we're in UJ's bedroom and one bedside lamp is on. This is the hour before bedtime, and it's important for melatonin to start to kick in. Now we're down to about 50 to 65 lux.

When measuring lux, even the low digits are meaningful. A Korean experiment found that young men who slumbered in 10-lux light for just one night had worse scores on working memory tests the next day than those who slept in 5-lux light. Their brain scans also showed lower-than-usual activation in an area associated with attention and control, the right frontal gyrus. The disturbing thing is they didn't realize that they were subtly impaired. (We're all less self-aware than we think.) Less melatonin is secreted, the researchers posit, which makes sleep shallower and more segmented. Without the mind's ability to juggle concepts and draw on memory, everything is harder: math, writing, directions, attention, you name it. Whether kids who sleep in low light also have attention or working memory issues is unexplored but not improbable, so why risk it? Aim for 5 lux of light or less while sleeping.

The only studies I found that address the impact of light on the structure of the developing brain are on rodents, but the outcome is troubling enough to flag. When rats slept in light as dim as 1 to 5 lux, scientists could see a change in the structure of neurons, specifically smaller dendrites, in the memory regions of the animals' brains. It seems that the light interferes with the structure of sleep and, in particular, the phase of sleep when "neural fertilizer," brain-derived neurotrophic factor (BDNF), is produced. The worst-case scenario here is that chronic exposure to dim light at night, including the light pollution from skyglow and streetlights, could cause long-term deficiencies in memory and concentration for young and old alike.

To conclude our routine:

- By 7:45 I rotate the face of my daughter's bedside clock so that only 1 lux lands on her pillow, and slip into bed next to her.

Only on nights like this, in the ember-like glow of the night-light, does a day fade out properly. UJ's eyes get soft and big. The cocoon of darkness and the rising melatonin offers the right mood and mindset for reflection and storytelling. Just as it did for the Lenape, as UJ would say—who, incidentally, had their own stories about light. One night I share with her the Lenape legend about the sun's origin. In summary, it goes like this:

> *The world became cold and dark. The people and animals panicked, for they missed the light and warmth. Rainbow Crow, a bird with bright multicolored plumage, bravely volunteered to ask the Creator for a source of light. The Creator agreed and gave Rainbow Crow a burning stick to carry home in his beak. As Crow flew through the heavens, the fire on that stick became the sun that lights up the world. But not without sacrifice! Poor Crow had carried the fiery light for too long, and that's why his voice is forever hoarse from being scorched, and his colorful feathers are forever charred.*

The legend, especially when spun out in its full glory, speaks to the power of light. We can't flourish without it. But we need to use it strategically, for even a little too much denies us our color and range. It can burn us out.

DECEMBER

All Is Calm, All Is Bright

*A new tool for an ancient resilience
and self-regulation trick*

IN THE ERA of the quantified self, you, like me, might look for ways to track and measure your efforts. I want to see evidence of improvement after subjecting my child to a year of experiments to support guts and grit and everything related: working memory, learning, sociability, creativity, willpower, and overall health and spirit. The subjective results are in (a great success, of course), but I want hard data. Patterns. Code. I yearn for numbers on a screen, showing an upward trend, a strong optimistic signal that cuts through the fog of doubt and uncertainty.

Nothing can measure everything, I know. But there is a tracker that can measure *something*, and it's a lot better than nothing for a megalomaniacal, results-driven parent. It's simple, nearby, reliable, and accurate to the moment.

This tracker is the ticker, the heartbeat.

Once upon a time I'd have thought that a heartbeat that remains steady and unvarying is a sign of strength. But to my surprise, cardiac consistency is the hobgoblin of weaker minds and bodies. "The stiffest tree is most easily cracked, while the bamboo or willow survives by bending with the wind," the martial artist Bruce Lee said. So it is with the heart, which you want to bend to the ever-changing circumstances of the nervous system rather than pump on robotically, oblivious of the state of body and mind. You want a heartbeat to be variable.

Heart rate variability (HRV) is a measure of irregularity in the intervals between beats. If you're curious about how resilient you and your kid are, at least physiologically (which in the end can't be separated from cognitively), you could do worse than to strap on a cheap, noninvasive heart monitor and download an app to measure your HRV. The subtle speed-up-slow-down between successive beats reveals more about resilience than does heart rate, which only counts the number of beats per minute. If the child has a heart rate of 120 beats per minute, she's stressed or excited—that's a no-brainer. With HRV, you also get a sense of how well she can respond to whatever's going on and how well she'll recover. A high HRV measurement is generally a sign of resilience: the ability to adapt to and bounce back from stresses. In that context, it's not much of a stretch to see how HRV is also linked with sociability, decision making, creativity, and problem solving.

HRV can be used in two ways: to monitor resilience and to improve it. After a year of experiments to trick out UJ's nervous system, there's something satisfying about using a tool that may reflect—and enhance—our humble efforts: the microbes, the bioflavonoids, the greenery, the touching, the storytelling, the magnesium, the weird exercises, everything.

So, how well did we do, how well are we doing, how good can we get? Beat by beat, being and becoming.

Nothing is, everything is becoming. —Heraclitus of Ephesus

UJ sits as still as possible, breathing steadily as my phone's camera turns her finger a delicate, glowing shell pink. We're taking her HRV reading. The number we'll see is not a true baseline: we recently flew through the freezing night to Barcelona, Spain, by way of a layover in Milan, where we crashed in an airport hotel before driving two hours to the city's smaller airport and boarding another plane. Well after midnight UJ and Ami were outside our Airbnb rental shouting *Hola!* to holiday revelers. Now it's the following afternoon, and I don't need the HRV reading to see that UJ's springs have sprung. But I want to see how badly.

A heart rate variability reading is easy, cheap, reliable, and non-invasive. Most of us already have a basic tool for the job: a smartphone like the one I'm using on UJ. There are dozens of apps that, in conjunction with a basic strap-on heart monitor, can measure the intervals between heartbeats. Some apps don't even require the strap, just a steady index finger placed over the lens (details to follow). When we feel lazy or spontaneous, like now, we use the smartphone camera without the strap.

Not long before I became pregnant with UJ, a developmental psychologist named Janet DiPietro, at Johns Hopkins University, published the sort of study that caught my eye. I was obsessed with prenatal predictors, and DiPietro found that fetal heart rate variability is a decent predictor of the baby's condition, maturity, and, in a sense, early potential. DiPietro found that a higher heart rate variability after twenty-eight weeks in the womb is linked with better behavioral outcomes in infancy and even up to age three, the oldest age group she tested. Fetuses with the highest HRV had markedly better language development and symbolic play in early toddlerhood than fetuses with low variability. They reached all their milestones sooner. Other research found that they're less likely to die from sudden infant death syndrome (SIDS).

Armed with this intel, I pressed the heart monitor to my bulging abdomen and cheered on fetal UJ's accelerations and decelerations as a sign of sentient life. I hadn't taken proper HRV measurements at the time, but my obstetrician commented on the variability of the beat. Whatever it was in there, it was no robot. Maybe it was no coincidence that UJ was early to reach the stages of puppet play and reading. That slightly irregular heart rhythm may have signaled promise. But why?

The explanation is rooted in the autonomic nervous system— the body's complex of nerves, blood vessels, hormones, and muscles. The autonomic system has two branches: the sympathetic and the parasympathetic. The sympathetic system is like a gas pedal. Think of the famous fight-or-flight response. Whenever a person is irritated, flustered, anxious, sick, bullied, overexerted, or otherwise pushed or pressed, the sympathetic system drives the heart to beat faster and with tick-tock regularity. (Stress out a pregnant woman too much, and she and her fetus both have faster heartbeats with less variability.) The sympathetic system is survivalist mode—it keeps us ticking steadily at an adrenaline-fueled eighty to one hundred fixed beats per minute (and kids' even higher), no matter what's going on, to get us through the ordeal. The prefrontal cortex basically goes offline and automatic processes take over. Problem is, too much of this puts us on the road to burnout.

The parasympathetic branch is the brakes of the operation. It sends a signal to the heart that says *Slow the heck down.* In every inhale the sympathetic dominates; but in every exhale the parasympathetic kicks in, and the strength of its pull back determines heart rate variability. The more pull, the higher the HRV. Looking at a monitor, you'd see the intervals jump around a lot. There might be 1.1 seconds between beats, then .9 seconds, then 1.2 seconds. That's what it looks like when the body is self-regulating in response to changes in the environment. And self-regulation, after all, is a cornerstone of learning.

You might be curious about where this parasympathetic pullback comes from, and how to strengthen it. Remember the vagus nerve that meanders between the brain stem and the digestive system by way of the heart, lungs, and kidneys? The one that gut microbes use to communicate with the brain? Signals that go *up* the vagus terminate at nucleus tractus solitarius, a switching station in the brain stem. From there, the signals travel to regions that produce neurotransmitters that subdue overexcited neurons. This has a calming effect on a person. Among the signals that travel *down* the vagus to the heart are those that release acetylcholine, a chemical brake. Acetylcholine slows down heart rate and varies the space between each beat, leading to higher HRV.

A little more than twenty years ago, a man named Stephen Porges, then director of the Brain-Body Center at the University of Illinois at Chicago, introduced a radical idea: the vagus nerve, he said, consists of two systems; the first freezes us up when we're afraid and the second regulates stress and social responses. Focusing on the second, he proposed that the stronger the vagal nerve activity, or vagal tone, the stronger the parasympathetic pull, and the more the heartrate decreases with each exhalation.

People with better vagal tone, Porges pointed out, are more relaxed because a stimulated vagus releases prolactin, oxytocin, vasopressin, and other calming hormones. It's no surprise, then, that they're better at responding in a controlled way to the ever-changing conditions around them. They have more grace under pressure. Vagus nerve signals, Porges noted, also suppress inflammatory cytokines that, over the long-term, may otherwise lead to depression and anxiety.

Porges's polyvagal theory spawned great interest in the vagus. Hundreds of studies later, the general consensus is that if there's a key to self-regulation, resilience, and health, it involves a well-strummed vagus nerve. Some research even suggests that the vagus triggers the body's ultimate act of resilience: the stimulation of stem cells to produce new cells that can repair worn-out organs, recover memory, and grow neurons. Name anything that's linked with resilience, and it touches on the vagus. One could argue that our resilience-building experiments, in a way, are all vagus nerve hacks:

- *Gut microbiome?* Check. The gut microbiome uses the vagus nerve to send signals to the brain. *Bifidobacterium* and *Lactobacillus* especially enhance vagal tone and are thought to reduce anxiety. Cut the vagus nerve, as researchers did in rats, and these probiotics no longer have a calming effect. (A worthwhile experiment would be to see if people with a more diverse microbiome or who take certain probiotics also have increased HRV and a stronger parasympathetic system in general. I have a hunch that they do.)
- *Nature?* Check. Walking in a forest, or even seeing pictures of nature, increases vagus nerve activity and HRV.
- *Magnesium?* Check. Magnesium deficiency, which afflicts most of us, reduces vagal nerve activity. Incidentally, a study on veterans found that those who ate green leafy vegetables, the highest in magnesium, also had the highest HRV. It's just a correlation, but an interesting one.
- *Flavonoids?* Check. Flavonoids in blueberries and other fruit and vegetables feed healthy gut bacteria such as *Lactobacillus* and *Bifidobacterium*. Flavonols, a class of flavonoids in fruits and vegetables, have also been shown to prevent inflammation of the vagus nerve.
- *Proprioceptive exercise?* Check. Proprioceptors, sensors everywhere in the body, send signals up the vagus nerve to the nucleus tractus solitarius in the brain, which in turn sends signals down the vagus back to the heart. Balance and motion exercises increase gut flow, which also stimulates the vagus. A small but very recent Finnish study of epileptic patients showed that stimulation of the

vagus nerve improves working memory significantly because it increases the stimulant norepinephrine in the neocortex, hippocampus, amygdala, and other parts of the brain. The theory is that this hormonal surge increases attention and helps us to focus on the information that working memory juggles.

- *Touch?* Check. Affectionate touch when willingly received—massaging, caressing, even a one-second resting of the hand—stimulates the vagus nerve to trigger oxytocin production. Oxytocin, the so-called bonding hormone, gives us that feeling of warm expansion in the chest when we're moved emotionally. Babies who have skin-to-skin contact have better vagal tone than those who don't, and also more mature neurodevelopment. They also have higher HRV.

- *Cognitive reappraisal?* Check. Cognitive reappraisal first requires an awareness of when the sympathetic nervous system kicks in—the racing heart, the sweaty palms, the butterflies—followed by activation of the parasympathetic nervous system, which is under the sway of our thinking. (*The butterflies in my stomach are helping me.*) Studies show that when people practice cognitive reappraisal, their HRV increases significantly more than when suppressing or ignoring a challenge, a sign of emotion regulation. People with low HRV are also more prone to intrusive bad thoughts.

- *Narrative reappraisal?* Check. Several studies found that when people translate their painful experiences into a story with a beginning, middle, and end, their HRV increases significantly. In the most recent experiment, led by researchers at the City University of New York, people who were instructed to write expressively about their academic anxieties as a story experienced an increase in HRV, especially if they prefer to process emotions through words, while those who wrote about neutral topics showed no such gains.

- *Lighting?* Check. Outdoor light increases vagal tone and HRV more than indoor light, and the quality and quantity of indoor light affects the vagus. Some studies show that when people spend a day under fluorescent lighting, their HRV is much lower at night than it is during a day under LED lights. Melatonin, meanwhile, reduces the sympathetic reflex. A Finnish study on ten- to fourteen-year-old kids found that the heaviest users of electronic screens at night have a lower HRV during the following school day. Screen glow interferes with their melatonin rise and parasympathetic recovery at night.

After a year of vagal toning, I hope to see UJ's HRV display on the smartphone screen look as jagged as the Swiss Alps we just flew over. The higher the variability, the stronger her resilience.

Heart rate variability is measured in milliseconds referred to as R-R (beat-to-beat) intervals. There are several different methods to calculate this, but the most accurate and relevant one used in studies for short-term HRV is called RMSSD, which, if you want to get technical, means the root-mean square differences of the successive beat-to-beat intervals. From previous readings, I knew that UJ's normal HRV (RMSSD) varies as much as 70 to 140 milliseconds (or 65–80 on the logged HRV 1–100 scale), which compares favorably to athletes in their twenties. This is not because UJ is an ironchild wunderkind. Kids generally have much higher HRV than adults, and many studies have found that the variability increases until a child is six to nine years old and then stabilizes in adolescence. (Physical fitness increases HRV. The older and more sedentary we get, the more vagal tone we lose.)

The problem with the smartphone app is that if you jerk your finger around too much or press too hard on the camera lens, the software can't parse the signal. That's UJ's problem this afternoon.

"Let me hold it for you," I say diplomatically. I take her index finger and press it on the device.

"No! I'll do it!" We tussle for control of the phone. She wins and doggedly sits still for the minute it takes to measure HRV.

On this travel day in Barcelona, UJ's HRV is more "mature" than I'd like to see: it's in the lower 70s (RMSSD), which puts her somewhere around the eightieth percentile for her age group, going by a Belgian study of children ages five to ten (see chart on page 235). She's jet-lagged, exasperated, sleep deprived, and put upon by maternal meddling—on her vacation, no less. As an indication of her fatigue, she has no interest in her number. I'll take it for now, but I've become something of a Tiger Mom for calm, clarity, and control. How can we do better?

Do not learn how to react. Learn how to respond. —Anonymous

If there's one thing I've learned when experimenting together with young kids, it's that you've got to make the effort compelling. To them. The flickering numbers on a smartphone mean little to nothing to a six-year-old. Boredom, annoyance, and pressure compromise heart rate variability and you get an off-reading. So, I switched tactics and focused on the "challenge."

It's called Buddha breath. I explain to UJ that "Buddha breath" is a way of breathing that she can do any time she feels stressed or overwhelmed or otherwise off-kilter. The idea is to sit or lie down and take in a deep breath. You breathe in a little slower than you do normally, through the nose, and breathe out with gentle force on the rib cage. (A six- to twelve-year-old normally takes twelve to twenty breaths a minute, one- to five-year-olds take twenty to thirty, on the lower end when relaxed. I want her to aim for ten breathes a minute or fewer.) This is mindful breathing, and she tells me she has learned something like this at school. *Try to breathe in for three seconds, breathe out for six. Repeat for a minute or two.*

To get a sense of the day's baseline, I strap a heart rate monitor around her chest (acquired for less than fifty dollars. See page 234 for details). I pair it with my smartphone app as she lies back and stares into space. HRV: 90 milliseconds (RMSSD).

"Now, Buddha breath!" I say.

She takes silly, shallow panting breaths. *Hee hee hee.*

"No," I say wearily. "If Buddha breathed like that, people would've been terrified of him. Inhale through your nose. Don't strain. Expand your rib cage. *Breathing in, 1-2-3. Breathing out, 1-2-3-4-5-6.* Hey, you're six! Breathe out six."

She tries again—1-2-3-4-5-6!—all in a rushing stream. More silliness, and I can feel my own HRV taking a nosedive.

I stay silent for a moment, focused on breathing out my irritation.

UJ finally speaks. "It's better when I put one hand on my stomach, Mama, and one hand on my chest."

The hippie kid is finally kicking in. This is a child whose New Year's resolution is to do more yoga on rooftops. She literally hugs trees. Earlier this month I took her to a mindfulness/meditation class, where we did mother-daughter exercises like move our chopsticks together, touching, in mirror synchronicity, and chewed an apple mindfully. She had a blast. Afterward she informed me, with complete earnestness, that she meditates best to a gong.

"Can you feel your diaphragm expand like a Buddha's? Can you feel the difference between filling your lungs and filling the space that's lower? Feel mine."

Slow, deep diaphragmatic breathing is thought to improve vagal tone in, well, a heartbeat. On the screen you can see the heart rate variability jump up. For UJ's little lungs, three seconds of inhale and six seconds of exhale feel just right. The exhale is when the parasympathetic branch kicks in, bringing down the heart rate while varying the time between successive heartbeats. The trick is the long exhale.

"This is something not everyone knows," I say to UJ in an excited whisper. "The exhale is where you get your center back." Never ever hold your breath when you're expecting a painful moment like a shot or when you're about to perform in front of your class and you feel anxious, I tell her. Always release it slowly. *Focus on your long exhale.* She nods seriously. If you ever hold your breath on the inhale, the sympathetic system takes over, and the anxiety is intensified. Your heart rate variability plummets.

UJ lies back and closes her eyes. Breathe in, breathe out *slowly*. Now I hear her taking in great heaving breaths, open-mouthed, like a guppy in slow motion. She's trying too hard. Maybe she's feeling pressured by me and this last crazy month of experimentation; her HRV is going down rather than up. She's annoyed that I'm correcting her. Her numbers bottom out at 40 (RMSSD), possibly her worst result ever.

Slowly. There are guided breathing apps that may help some (think: a circle expanding and contracting), but they don't help UJ. She finds the graphics and the pneumatic breathing sounds distracting and disturbing. But after a few minutes she lands on her own technique, which she tells me she picked up from a book. While listening to her breath she homes in on small background noises, real or imagined—the leaves rustling, a distant bird, the feathery wind. She finds her center. I know she's not faking it when her face takes on a look of utter absorption.

A number of studies focusing on athletes have found that when people tracked their HRV as they breathed, as a form of biofeedback (about six breaths/minute), their performance escalated dramatically. Their stress levels during subsequent competition diminished dramatically and their reaction times sped up. (In some studies, subjects practiced breathing at home every day for twenty minutes, which may be a stretch.) Awareness is key. If a six-year-old, or an eleven-year-old, could do Buddha breath automatically whenever she feels overwhelmed, barely noticing the switch in modes, how fortunate that child would be in life.

Whether six-breaths-a-minute Buddha breathing can be cultivated as an automatic unconscious habit for any kid (or adult) remains to be proven. The general consensus is that it is possible, in theory, with extensive practice at times of high stress. It takes conditioning—start by consciously doing this type of breathing every time a frustrating, tense, or scary situation pops up. A kid's knee-jerk reaction to stress would need to be the slow ebb and flow of the mindful inhale and the slower, deeper exhale.

Inhale, exhale . . . In this moment, UJ is in the groove. I start measuring again, and let the heartbeart monitor roll for two minutes. Her heart rate variability begins to trend upward.

This time her RMSSD is a soaring 120 milliseconds. In this moment, she's at the tip-top of her age group.

In this moment.

Biohack: Hacking the HRV

The body reacts to everything: exercise, emotions, observations, situations, one's own nervous energy and that of others. How well does it respond? How well does it rebound? Neither pulse nor blood pressure measures resilience, but heart rate variability—the difference in time, in milliseconds, between successive heartbeats— does. An easy, reliable, and inexpensive way to measure HRV—in just one or two minutes—is with smartphone apps. At the time of printing, there are four apps that we use regularly: HRV4Training, Camera HRV, Elite HRV, and HRV+. The first two apps involve putting a finger on the lens of a smartphone camera; the latter require a Bluetooth-communicating heart monitor (popular choices are manufactured by Polar and Garmin), which costs as little as forty-five dollars. We've used both methods and the results are similar. When taking measurements:

• Keep still. Movement throws off the results.
• Be aware that taking a measurement while lying down results in a higher HRV than sitting. Standing up yields the lowest HRV results.

- When comparing daily results, be consistent with your measurements by using the same time of day, the same posture, and the same breathing pattern.
- Both distressing and exciting moments can decrease HRV. When measuring, take the child's emotions into account.

Many apps score heart rate variability logarithmically using their own scale (often from 1–100) based on a measure called RMSSD (the square root of the mean squared differences of successive R-R intervals greater than 50 milliseconds). These apps also report the raw RMSSD, which is helpful when comparing your child's scores to the average for his or her age group. The following HRV data come from a study of 460 children, ages five through ten, using a chest strap heart monitor while lying down.

Percentile values for RMSSD (ms) by age and gender*

Age	Percentile (Boys)						Percentile (Girls)				
	2.5	25th	50th	75th	97.5th		2.5	25th	50th	75th	97.5th
5	26	39	50	64	112		14	40	55	71	107
6	35	61	80	105	181		12	39	55	74	117
7	27	57	77	103	175		14	43	62	85	141
8	19	48	68	92	152		17	47	68	93	159
9	21	52	74	99	164		22	51	72	97	166
10	27	61	84	112	184		27	54	72	96	160

In adolescence heart rate variability begins to decline, and the extent depends on stress and physical fitness. For unathletic teenage girls, the median RMSSD is 69 ms (49 for 25th percentile; 100 at

25th percentile, 88 at the 75th percentile). For athletic teenage girls the median is 95 ms (77 at the 25th percentile, 119 at the 75th percentile). For athletic teenage boys, the median is 78 ms (78 at 25th percentile, 125 at the 75th percentile).* For adults, there is tremendous variability in the RMSSD, but most thirty-five- to fifty-year-olds fall within 50 to 70 ms.

Experiment with HRV as a way to track resilience daily. Athletes, professional speakers, and fans of the quantified life use HRV in training daily to control their stress response and bounce back after frustrations, challenges, and threats. Measured in the morning, HRV may also predict how the day may go—how well a person will deal with adversity. When HRV is below baseline, some people see it as a sign to slow down and take it easy. When it's up, they push themselves harder, taking the result as a sign that it's a good day to perform or to compete.

My favorite way to use HRV with a child is to increase resilience on the fly by using a tracker as a biofeedback tool. There are many ways to deliberately dial down the sympathetic nervous system and stimulate the vagus in the short and long term:

- moderate aerobic exercise or intense exercise (it often causes a temporary decrease in HRV followed by an increase)
- chanting and yoga
- taking a cold shower or simply immersing the face in cold water (a surprise, but it activates the body's response, including production of thyroid activating hormone, to bring one back to the stable middle)
- inflammation-reducing diet with an emphasis on leafy greens
- reduced stress
- foot massage or other intimate contact
- lying on your right side

- Buddha breath
- any activity that puts one in a state of "flow," a state of feeling fully immersed and engaged

Buddha breath is our name for a heart-rate-variability-and-resilience-building skill that can be cultivated with daily practice. It's a variant of diaphragmatic breathing, or pranayama, the yogic practice of slowing and extending the breaths. To develop a habit, challenge your child to spend five to ten minutes practicing deep breathing every day for six weeks. The inhale should be deep but "effortless." Exhale for longer than the inhale (this is when the parasympathetic system kicks in).

Have your child place his hand on his belly and feel his stomach and lower back go concave with the exhale and expand for each inhale. Using a heart rate monitor as a biofeedback tool, the kid learns how to modify her breathing so that her numbers climb as her parasympathetic reflexes kick in. (Some apps guide breathing [Elite HRV] or provide a digital landscape [BioZen] in which features pop up when the user reaches certain physiological thresholds.) In time, Buddha breath may become a habit, and the child will no longer need to use a device. The awareness of the heart's rhythms combined with the ability to control them—that's wisdom and power.

* Sources: N. Michaels, et al., "Determinants and Reference Values of Short-Term Heart Rate Variability in Children," *European Journal of Applied Physiology* 113, no. 6 (June 2013): 1477–88; Vivek Kumar Sharma, et al., "Heart Rate Variability in Adolescents—Normative Data Stratified by Sex and Physical Activity," *Journal of Clinical and Diagnostic Research* 9, no. 10 (October 2015): CC08–CC13.

The better the Buddha breath, the more Buddha-like the breather. We're not all equals when it comes to deep abdominal exhales or any vagal-tone-boosting activity. A research group at the Max Planck Institute in Germany hypothesized that the people who do it easily and instinctively are friendlier and more generous than the norm. After all, virtuous traits require self-regulation, and anyone who automatically controls his or her breathing and heart rate variability under pressure has what it takes.

To test their idea, the researchers challenged a group of volunteers to a biofeedback task in which they had to reach a desired mind-body state to raise a ball on a screen. If a person exceeded an HRV threshold, the red spinning ball would rise. No one told the volunteers to use their Buddha breath, observation of the body, or any other technique to raise their HRV. Some did it naturally, as if they'd been controlling their hearts all their lives, and this group fascinated the researchers. Were these the people, they wondered, who'd put a coin in a beggar's hat or stop the elevator door from closing to let in one more rider?

To find out, all the volunteers were given hypothetical scenarios in which they had money and could spend it, or not. Would they give it away charitably? Or would they maximize individual gain over group gain? How much did they favor an even distribution of wealth versus payouts only to people close to them? Were they purely generous, or did they only part with money when they expected something in return or when paying back those who helped them?

A pattern emerged, and with it a confirmation of the researchers' hypothesis. The people who were good at raising their HRV on demand were indeed the same ones who gave away a fair amount of their money, and not merely out of social norms like reciprocity or punishment. Their generosity was motivated by altruism. You could say it came from the heart.

Other studies have found that you can predict compassion by looking at people's heart rate variability. People who have an HRV upsurge when they see, for instance, suffering kittens or homeless people are more altruistic and willing to donate their money to a charity for the cause. People who maintain a higher-than-average HRV when hearing about sick children are more willing to share resources with them. In these cases, a high HRV is a sure sign of emotional responsiveness.

Think for a moment about why this might be. We know that high HRV is a triumph of the parasympathetic, the branch of the nervous system that increases a sense of calm. The vagus nerve is stimulated, which has the knock-on effect of a slower heart rate and respiration. This in turn redirects energy to other processes like social awareness and flexibility. (A faster heart rate, in contrast, activates the amygdala, which further primes the fear and anger response.) The vagus nerve also influences the release of oxytocin, the so-called calm-and-connect hormone.

Kids generally have much better vagal tone than adults, but there's still a very wide spectrum. Psychologists at the University of California Davis wondered if preschoolers who have strong vagal tone would turn out to be more caring and empathetic years later than those with weaker tone. They launched a long-run experiment that began with a pool of three- and four-year-olds, each of whom was tested for vagal tone (using an HRV marker called respiratory sinus arrhythmia).

In the first stage of the experiment the kids witnessed an accident: an adult dropping everything in her arms as she fell and hurt herself. Which kids said, "Oh no!"? Which ones asked if she was OK? Which ones turned away, unmoved and expressionless, and went back to their toys? Behind-the-scenes experimenters rated each preschooler's level of empathic concern. Can you guess which kids scored highest?

The children with strong vagal tone and high HRV, just as the researchers hypothesized. These kids noticed distress in others and empathized without being overwhelmed or threatened. They also perceived themselves as having more supportive friends. They had fewer adjustment problems, while those with poor vagal tone tended to be inhibited in new social situations and dislike novelty. Other studies show that the very act of giving and bonding strengthens vagal tone, which perpetuates a virtuous cycle.

What's surprising to note is that the children in the study with the strongest empathic response had strong vagal tone, but not the *strongest*. There was a threshold over which kids with the highest HRV were *less* sympathetic than average. Why? At a certain point, people may be able to control their emotions so well that they're capable of inhibiting feelings of personal distress or empathy for others.

Now, fast-forward five years, and the preschoolers in the UC Davis study are in third and fourth grades. The researchers could finally address their burning questions. Did the toddlers with the fairly strong vagal tone became more caring and sociable eight-year-olds compared to those with low vagal tone? Is heart rate variability in early childhood predictive of later behavior?

The answer is . . . yes. Generally speaking, the preschoolers with strong vagal tone became grade-schoolers whose moms and teachers gave them high marks for comforting others in pain or volunteering to help. On the whole they were more sensitive to others in class and likelier to compliment their peers than were kids with low vagal tone. They were likelier to stick up for a kid who was being bullied. Other studies show that children with strong vagal tone are less defensive when confronted by a frenemy or a dilemma or an intrusive albeit well-intended parent or, later, a romantic partner—all because their sympathetic fight-or-flight reflexes aren't trigger-ready. They can control their own distress or anxiety more easily, which allows them to turn their attention outward.

One study found that people with high HRV even *look* more generous and approachable, as if you could pick them out in a crowd. (The vagus regulates muscles in the face and head, which is why you can tell from voice or expression if a person is stressed.) Or maybe they'll pick you. An Australian study found that people with a high resting HRV are likelier to affiliate and favor others in a group more strongly than those with a low HRV even if that group is just a clutch of strangers who share a preference for the same art. HRV is a sign of not just physiological adaptability but also social adaptability.

The best news is that HRV can be consciously raised in the same way as awareness. Over the past year—and perhaps I can credit our interventions—UJ has become more compassionate and aware of human suffering and more sociable generally. She's become a bleeding heart about the environment and children's rights (the sly sprite). She wants to give Manhattan back to the Lenape and restore the island to its previous state of forests and streams. She lectures bus drivers for idling and ice cream truck vendors for spewing out poisonous exhaust. Much of this new behavior is no doubt maturity: a six-year-old is more outward-looking now than she was when younger. But it's also a sign of health, focus, and resilience. Could this emergence of passionate activism be raising her heart rate variability, or is it a reflection of it?

The likely answer is both. It's another virtuous cycle.

It is only about things that do not interest one that one can give a really unbiased opinion. —Oscar Wilde

In recent years, some buffs of polyvagal theory started to get bigger, headier ideas. If heart rate variability can predict who has resilience, self-control, sensitivity, and empathy, they reasoned, then why not go further? Maybe you could use HRV to predict who has the ultimate virtue of all: wisdom. Solomon-esque wisdom—the ability to make unbiased judgments, not just clever ones.

A case could be made. The link between heart rate variability and self-control was well-established. More than a dozen studies found that people with higher-than-average HRV show more activity in the areas of the brain that give rise to executive function: planning, paying attention, inhibiting irrelevant thoughts, reasoning, and problem-solving. The most vagally toned bounce back faster from anger, so they might not let their emotions get the best of them. They have a stronger working memory, so they can juggle several ideas in the mind at once, so they might be less hung up on one idea. They're better at squelching intrusive irrelevant thoughts. On a physiological level, they redirect energy to higher cognitive functions instead of frittering it all on simple sympathetic processes like a racing heart and intrusive thoughts.

All that probably adds up to wisdom, right? It seems to be a safe assumption anyway, so Igor Grossmann, a psychologist at Canada's University of Waterloo, decided to test it. Grossmann and two colleagues pooled together nearly two hundred participants (all adults) and asked them to identify a political and social issue relevant to society from a list that included environment/climate change, politics, health care, the economy, and other issues. Each person's heart rate variability was measured before and after the experiment.

The trio encouraged their subjects to think about the future and randomly assigned them to one of two perspectives: a first-person perspective, in which they were told to "immerse themselves" in a situation, or a self-distanced one in which they were told to "focus on" the situation. In each condition they had to address how the issue will unfold in the future and why.

Next, judges who were blind to the purpose of the experiment coded and rated each participant's response. Who recognized other people's points of view? Who searched for a compromise? How well, in the self-distanced exercise, could a person separate from his or her impassioned opinions and offer balance and insight?

The exercise here is too complex for a six-year-old, but I thought I'd try it anyway on UJ with a topic that she cares about: climate change. We're about to embark on a new year and have the future of the world to ponder. The golden moment after a Buddha breath session seems a good time for serious contemplation.

"The environment," I say. "Can you talk about it? How do you think this climate change problem is going to play out in the future? What will happen? Why do you think it's going to go that way?"

The sun has set, and the honking of cars outside sounds like foghorns.

After a minute she speaks. "I'm worried about Earth and all its problems," she says. "I want to go to another planet that's beautiful, like the ones in Ami's book [*Regards to the Man in the Moon* by Ezra Jack Keats]. It's good to have a choice. But it doesn't seem fair to leave behind all the plants and animals on Earth."

In the real study, every response was coded and rated by professionals who weren't the subjects' biased mamas. The more objective and inclusive of the other side's point of view, the higher the rating. So, what was it? Did people with a higher HRV offer wiser, better-balanced, and more insightful perspective than those with low HRV scores?

Not necessarily, it turns out. High-HRV types gave wiser responses than those who had low HRV, but *only* when they were explicitly instructed to self-distance themselves. They had to be primed. When talking about themselves in the first person as it related to an issue they cared about, they were just as likely to fall into an ego trap as anyone else. It didn't occur to most people to reason or balance their perspective, or describe the other side's perspective and then explain, objectively, why it's flawed. This isn't to say there weren't exceptions. When the researchers looked at all the wise, Solomon-esque statements in the study, whether made from a first-person or a third-person perspective, the top 20 percent were made by people with high heart rate variability, but it wasn't a significant number.

If there's a lesson here, it's this. Having a high HRV is linked to better judgment and insight, but only if a person consciously *chooses* to be impartial or is directed to think that way. Otherwise, high HRV types lapse into egocentric biases too, just like anyone else, or worse when they use their cognitive powers to strengthen a bubble world-view. Case in point: A study of stock market traders found that the best and most experienced profit maximizers are those with the highest heart rate variability. They may be able to control their emotions when making decisions, but not their self-interest.

Life is a process of becoming, a combination of states we have to go through. Where people fail is that they wish to elect a state and remain in it. This is a kind of death. —Anaïs Nin

On a practical level, it's not how favorably one's own heart rate variability compares to the average that matters. It's one's own baseline that's most instructive—that is, the day-to-day or even moment-to-moment variations. Many people test themselves every morning. There's a logic to this: you get a sense of where your body and mind are before the day begins. (I personally test in the morning and have found the result to be generally predictive of my energy levels throughout the day.)

But taking a minute in the morning isn't always practical with children. UJ tests herself before bed, and the results are something of a barometer of the day that passed. A number below her baseline might signal that she's off: fighting an illness or fatigue, or that she's troubled about something, overexerted or overstimulated. (Physical exertion can drive HRV down temporarily; over the long term, exercise elevates HRV.) Lower-than-normal results can be a cue to stop and check in. What's wrong? My daughter's heart rate variability always goes up when we tell a story together, or chat about dream houses or something else that transcends practicalities and engages the imagination. She has started to learn to breathe to slow down her heart rate and see her HRV climb. She has started to develop better body awareness.

The bonus: heart rate variability is linked with sleep quality. The higher the HRV during the day, the less time it takes to fall asleep, and the less likely the sleeper is to wake up during the night. (This makes evolutionary sense, for if our ancestors felt anxious or threatened by potential enemies that might attack at night, light sleep would serve them better.) But deep sleep is preferable, which shows up the next morning as higher heart rate variability. It's resilience building on resilience.

All of this is achievable (even preferable) without a gadget that reduces resilience to a number. I think of the HRV apps as a gateway tool to biohacking, which in turn leads to more body awareness. Maybe someday she won't need the device. When UJ gets too brittle and bombastic, I want her to feel how that behavior affects her body. My hope—my master plan—is for her and her sister (eventually) to develop enough mind-body awareness to regulate themselves reflexively. May they someday feel the tightness in their chests or the butterflies of stress and learn to adjust their minds and bodies to maximize the stimulation (cognitive reappraisal) and release the unhealthy stress.

UJ's first week after winter break is stormy. She doesn't win a trophy in a school chess match. (*You didn't really expect to win if you don't play in your free time anymore, right?*) She has a performance in which she expertly plays a Lenape girl, which is exhilarating but still fraught. (Excitement, too, takes an emotional toll and reduces HRV.) During her Friday violin lesson she struggles to play a duet in sync. (*You were spacing out, sweetie.*) This is life, right? But by the end of this week even a normally resilient kid would lose some spring, so when little Ami pulls UJ's hair and pinches her for the umpteenth time, she snaps. She kicks.

"Time out!" I say, pointing to the couch.

"No! It's Friday!" she protests. "We're watching a movie!"

"Not unless you recenter yourself."

"Only if I can use the thing with the strap!" she shouts. She wants to measure her HRV—it's a fun time out—but only on her own terms. I suspect that she also likes the feeling of control when she watches her breath change her numbers. So, she wins. I make a big show of sighing as I strap the wireless heart monitor around her winter-pale, skinny chest, and record her HRV with two different apps (Elite HRV and HRV+) in succession. Then I hug her.

She lies there, in the dim light, breathing in, 1-2-3-4. Breathing out, 1-2-3-4-5-6. ("Make sure your belly goes up and down, not your lungs," I whisper.) A dog barks. A siren wails. Ami pulls a toy alligator around the room, shouting, "In September for a while, I will ride a crocodile!" repeatedly, at top volume.

Through this, UJ breathes and her HRV rises: 90, 92, 94 . . . The better her vagal tone, the faster she'll rebound from stress. She has been complaining of a headache, and I'll hear no more about it after Buddha breath.

But Buddha breath can be challenging to maintain after a few minutes, so when her HRV is around 100 milliseconds, UJ turns away and reaches for her book. I'm now alone with the screen, and, it's interesting, I see her HRV climbing higher than it did before with deep breathing. Reading, it seems, puts her in a flow state, and heart rate variability is buoyant in moments of flow. Her numbers go up and up: 110, 120 . . .

The higher her heart rate variability, the more unpredictable the space between beats. The reel resembles an irregular landscape. Every dip, every peak, is a little bit different from the one before. If I were to graph a year in a child's life, a beat representing each day, it'd look a lot like this readout. Ups and downs, highs and lows. In some apps you'll see a target breathing pattern to help users achieve optimal results. The goal, it seems, is to reach some vagal-platonic ideal of responsiveness and resilience. How close can one get to that pin-nacle—for a minute, a day, a year, a lifetime?

I watch the kid's ragged heart rate variability numbers roll out on the screen. It's an ever-changing, responsive, chaotic, human pattern. It beats on and on, push-pull-faster-slower, with gorgeous irregularity, perfectly imperfect by its very nature.

Acknowledgments

T HIS BOOK ON wits, guts, and grit wouldn't be possible if I hadn't had an accomplice willing to be witty, gutsy, and gritty. That person is my daughter Una Joy. With her by my side, I had ample opportunities to experiment with the ideas in the book and to see how and to what extent they might apply to real life. I like to think that she had as much fun as I did—and developed a curiosity for science to boot. Her little sister, Amandine, played the perfect supporting role: solid eater, happy guinea pig, comic relief.

In writing this book I've drawn on the wisdom of hundreds of studies, and I'm indebted to the many researchers behind those studies. In particular, I would like to thank Tracy and Ross Alloway, Bettina Pause, Jasper Groot, Christopher Lowry, Kelly Ramirez, James Pennebaker, James Scott, and Claire Williams for their insights and for answering my random questions.

Many thanks go to my editor at Chicago Review Press, Lisa Reardon, who saw something in this book when it was just a seed of an idea and nurtured it through the publishing process. I'm grateful to Ellen Hornor, project editor extraordinare, for her incisive queries and patience with my fussy updates, and to Michelle Williams for her copyedit. Thanks also go to CRP's marketing manager, Mary Kravenas, for all her efforts in getting the word out.

Finally, I wish to thank my husband, Peter, for his support as I wrote this book and for his tolerance of our wacky family experiments as well as his ongoing contributions as yogurt chef. While the text ostensibly covers a year of our lives, the actual research and editing took much longer, and I'll always be grateful for those morning coffees and mugs of our favorite black orchid tea. The book is finished, Peter, Una Joy, and Ami! You survived it, and that itself is a show of resilience.

Selected Sources

Introduction

Duckworth, Angela L., Christopher Peterson, Michael D. Matthews, and Dennis R. Kelly. "Grit: Perseverance and Passion for Long-Term Goals." *Journal of Personality and Social Psychology* 92, no. 6 (June 2007): 1087–1101. http://doi .org/10.1037/0022-3514.92.6.1087.

Harms, P. D. "Angela Duckworth. Grit: The Power of Passion and Perseverance. New York, NY: Scribner, 2016, 352 pages, $28.00 hardcover." *Personnel Psychology* 69, no. 4 (2016): 1021–1024. http://doi.org/10.1111/peps.12198.

January: Does Grit Depend on Guts?

Allen, A. P., W. Hutch, Y. E. Borre, P. J. Kennedy, A. Temko, G. Boylan, E. Murphy, J. F. Cryan, T. G. Dinan, and G. Clarke. "*Bifidobacterium longum* 1714 as a Translational Psychobiotic: Modulation of Stress, Electrophysiology and Neurocognition in Healthy Volunteers." *Translational Psychiatry* 6, no. 11 (November 2016): e939. http://doi.org/10.1038/tp.2016.191.

Bercik, Premysl, Emmanuel Denou, Josh Collins, Wendy Jackson, Jun Lu, Jennifer Jury, Yikang Deng, Patricia Blennerhassett, Joseph Macri, Kathy D. McCoy, Elena F. Verdu, and Stephen M. Collins. "The Intestinal Microbiota Affect Central Levels of Brain-Derived Neurotropic Factor and Behavior in Mice." *Gastroenterology* 141, no. 2 (August 2011): 599–609–609.e1–3. http://doi .org/10.1053/j.gastro.2011.04.052.

Cryan, John F., and Timothy G. Dinan. "Mind-Altering Microorganisms: The Impact of the Gut Microbiota on Brain and Behaviour." *Nature Reviews Neuroscience* 13, no. 10 (October 2012): 701–712. http://doi.org/10.1038/nrn3346.

Dinan, Timothy G., and John F. Cryan. "Gut Instincts: Microbiota as a Key Regulator of Brain Development, Ageing and Neurodegeneration." *Journal of Physiology* 595, no. 2 (January 15, 2017): 489–503. http://doi.org/10.1113/JP273106.

Erny, Daniel, Anna Lena Hrabě de Angelis, Diego Jaitin, Peter Wieghofer, Ori Staszewski, Eyal David, and Hadas Keren-Shaul, et al. "Host Microbiota Constantly Control Maturation and Function of Microglia in the CNS." *Nature Neuroscience* 18, no. 7 (June 1, 2015): 965–977. http://doi.org/10.1038/nn.4030.

Gonçalves, Ana Teresa, Masashi Maita, Kunihiko Futami, Masato Endo, and Takayuki Katagiri. "Effects of a Probiotic Bacterial *Lactobacillus rhamnosus* Dietary Supplement on the Crowding Stress Response of Juvenile Nile Tilapia *Oreochromis niloticus*." *Fisheries Science* 77, no. 4 (May 27, 2011): 633–642. http://doi.org/10.1007/s12562-011-0367-2.

Jašarević, E., Ali B. Rodgers, and Tracy L. Bale. "A Novel Role for Maternal Stress and Microbial Transmission in Early Life Programming and Neurodevelopment." *Neurobiology of Stress* 1 (January 2015): 81–88. http://doi.org/10.1016/j.ynstr.2014.10.005.

Kato-Kataoka, A., K. Nishida, M. Takada, K. Suda, M. Kawai, K. Shimizu, and A. Kushiro, et al. "Fermented Milk Containing *Lactobacillus casei* Strain Shirota Prevents the Onset of Physical Symptoms in Medical Students under Academic Examination Stress." *Beneficial Microbes* 7, no. 2 (2016): 153–156. http://doi.org/10.3920/BM2015.0100.

Miller, Andrew H., Ebrahim Haroon, Charles L. Raison, and Jennifer C. Felger. "Cytokine Targets in the Brain: Impact on Neurotransmitters and Neurocircuits." *Depression and Anxiety* 30, no. 4 (March 6, 2013): 297–306. http://doi.org/10.1002/da.22084.

Mudd, Austin, Kirsten Berding, Mei Wang, Sharon M. Donovan, and Ryan N. Dilger. "Serum Cortisol Mediates the Relationship Between Fecal *Ruminococcus* and Brain N-Acetylaspartate in the Young Pig." *Gut Microbes* (July 13, 2017): 1–12. http://dx.doi.org/10.1080/19490976.2017.1353849.

Rao, A. Venket, Alison C. Bested, Tracey M. Beaulne, Martin A. Katzman, Christina Iorio, John M. Berardi, and Alan C. Logan. "A Randomized, Double-

Blind, Placebo-Controlled Pilot Study of a Probiotic in Emotional Symptoms of Chronic Fatigue Syndrome." *Gut Pathogens* 1, no. 1 (March 19, 2009): 6. http://doi.org/10.1186/1757-4749-1-6.

Rodríguez, Juan Miguel, Kiera Murphy, Catherine Stanton, R. Paul Ross, Olivia I. Kober, Nathalie Juge, and Ekaterina Avershina, et al. "The Composition of the Gut Microbiota Throughout Life, with an Emphasis on Early Life." *Microbial Ecology in Health and Disease* 26, no. 1 (February 2, 2015): 26050. http://doi.org/10.3402/mehd.v26.26050.

Savignac, H. M., B. Kiely, T. G. Dinan, and J. F. Cryan. "*Bifidobacteria* Exert Strain-Specific Effects on Stress-Related Behavior and Physiology in BALB/c Mice." *Neurogastroenterology and Motility* 26, no. 11 (November 2014): 1615–1627. http://doi.org/10.1111/nmo.12427.

Savignac, H. M., M. Tramullas, B. Kiely, T. G. Dinan, J. F. Cryan. "Bifidobacteria Modulate Cognitive Processes in an Anxious Mouse Strain." *Behavioural Brain Research* 287 (July 1, 2015): 59–72. http://doi.org/10.1016/j.bbr.2015.02.044.

Tillisch, Kirsten, Jennifer Labus, Lisa Kilpatrick, Zhiguo Jiang, Jean Stains, Bahar Ebrat, Denis Guyonnet, Sophie Legrain–Raspaud, Beatrice Trotin, Bruce Naliboff, and Emeran A. Mayer. "Consumption of Fermented Milk Product with Probiotic Modulates Brain Activity." *Gastroenterology* 144, no. 7 (June 2013): 1394–1401.e4. http://doi.org/10.1053/j.gastro.2013.02.043.

Turroni, Francesca, Elena Foroni, Paola Pizzetti, Vanessa Giubellini, Angela Ribbera, Paolo Merusi, and Patrizio Cagnasso, et al. "Exploring the Diversity of the Bifidobacterial Population in the Human Intestinal Tract." *Applied and Environmental Microbiology* 75, no. 6 (2009): 1534–1545. http://doi.org/10.1128/AEM.02216-08.

Turroni, Francesca, Clelia Peano, Daniel A. Pass, Elena Foroni, Marco Severgnini, Marcus J. Claesson, Colm Kerr, Jonathan Hourihane, Deirdre Murray, and Fabio Fuligni, et al. "Diversity of Bifidobacteria Within the Infant Gut Microbiota." *PloS One* 7, no. 5 (May 11, 2012): e36957. http://doi.org/10.1371/journal.pone.0036957.

Zijlmans, Maartje A. C., Katri Korpela, J. Marianne Riksen-Walraven, Willem M. de Vos, and Carolina de Weerth. "Maternal Prenatal Stress Is Associated with the Infant Intestinal Microbiota." *Psychoneuroendocrinology* 53 (March 2015): 233–245. http://doi.org/10.1016/j.psyneuen.2015.01.006.

February: On Gut Bugs and Social Butterflies

Buffington, Shelly A., Gonzalo Viana Di Prisco, Thomas A. Auchtung, Nadim J. Ajami, Joseph F. Petrosino, and Mauro Costa-Mattioli. "Microbial Reconstitution Reverses Maternal Diet-Induced Social and Synaptic Deficits in Offspring." *Cell* 165, no. 7 (June 16, 2016): 1762–1775. http://doi.org/10.1016/j.cell.2016.06.001.

Christian, Lisa M., Jeffrey D. Galley, Erinn M. Hade, Sarah Schoppe-Sullivan, Claire Kamp Dush, and Michael T. Bailey. "Gut Microbiome Composition Is Associated with Temperament During Early Childhood." *Brain, Behavior, and Immunity* 45 (March 2015): 118–127. http://doi.org/10.1016/j.bbi.2014.10.018.

Cryan, John F., and Timothy G. Dinan. "Mind-Altering Microorganisms: The Impact of the Gut Microbiota on Brain and Behaviour." *Nature Reviews Neuroscience* 13, no. 10 (October 2012): 701–712. http://doi.org/10.1038/nrn3346.

Desbonnet, L., G. Clarke, F. Shanahan, T. G. Dinan, and J. F. Cryan. "Microbiota Is Essential for Social Development in the Mouse." *Molecular Psychiatry* 19, no. 2 (2014): 146–148. http://doi.org/10.1038/mp.2013.65.

Dinan, Timothy G., Roman M. Stilling, Catherine Stanton, and John F. Cryan. "Collective Unconscious: How Gut Microbes Shape Human Behavior." *Journal of Psychiatric Research* 63 (April 2015): 1–9. http://doi.org/10.1016/j.jpsychires.2015.02.021.

Erdman, Susan E. "Microbes, Oxytocin, and Healthful Longevity." *Journal of Probiotics & Health* 2 (2014): 117. http://doi.org/10.4172/2329-8901.1000117.

Erdman, S. E., and T. Poutahidis. "Microbes and Oxytocin: Benefits for Host Physiology and Behavior." *International Review of Neurobiology* 131 (2016): 91–126. http://doi.org/10.1016/bs.irn.2016.07.004.

Meadow, James F., Adam E. Altrichter, Ashley C. Bateman, Jason Stenson, GZ Brown, Jessica L. Green, and Brendan J.M. Bohannan. "Humans Differ in Their Personal Microbial Cloud." *PeerJ* 3, no. 5 (September 22, 2015): e1258. http://doi.org/10.7717/peerj.1258.

Neuman, Hadar, Justine W. Debelius, Rob Knight, and Omry Koren. "Microbial Endocrinology: The Interplay Between the Microbiota and the Endocrine System." *FEMS Microbiology Reviews* 39, no. 4 (July 1, 2015): 509–521. http://doi.org/10.1093/femsre/fuu010.

O'Mahony, S. M., G. Clarke, T. G. Dinan, and J. F. Cryan. "Early-Life Adversity and Brain Development: Is the Microbiome a Missing Piece of the Puzzle?" *Neuroscience* 342 (2017): 37–54. http://doi.org/10.1016/j.neuroscience.2015.09.068.

Sonnenburg, Erica D., Samuel A. Smits, Mikhail Tikhonov, Steven K. Higginbottom, Ned S. Wingreen, and Justin L. Sonnenburg. "Diet-Induced Extinctions in the Gut Microbiota Compound over Generations." *Nature* 529, no. 7585 (January 14, 2016): 212–215. http://doi.org/10.1038/nature16504.

Stilling, Roman M., Seth R. Bordenstein, Timothy G. Dinan, and John F. Cryan. "Friends with Social Benefits: Host-Microbe Interactions as a Driver of Brain Evolution and Development?" *Frontiers in Cellular and Infection Microbiology* 4, no. 46 (October 29, 2014): 147. http://doi.org/10.3389/fcimb .2014.00147.

Tian, Gang, Xiying Wu, Daiwen Chen, Bing Yu, and Jun He. "Adaptation of Gut Microbiome to Different Dietary Nonstarch Polysaccharide Fractions in a Porcine Model." *Molecular Nutrition & Food Research* (July 18, 2017): 1700012. http://doi.org/10.1002/mnfr.201700012.

Turroni, Francesca, Elena Foroni, Paola Pizzetti, Vanessa Giubellini, Angela Ribera, Paolo Merusi, and Patrizio Cagnasso, et al. "Exploring the Diversity of the Bifidobacterial Population in the Human Intestinal Tract." *Applied and Environmental Microbiology* 75, no. 6 (March 2009): 1534–1545. http://doi .org/10.1128/AEM.02216-08.

Turroni, Silvia, Jessica Fiori, Simone Rampelli, Stephanie L. Schnorr, Clarissa Consolandi, Monica Barone, and Elena Biagi, et al. "Fecal Metabolome of the Hadza Hunter-Gatherers: A Host-Microbiome Integrative View." *Scientific Reports* 6, no. 1 (2016): 32826. http://doi.org/10.1038/srep32826.

March: Let Them Eat Mudcakes

Bowers, S. J., C. J. Olker, E. Song, K. P. Wright, M. Fleshner, C. A. Lowry, M. H. Vitaterna, and F. W. Turek. "0146 Immunization with Heat-Killed Mycobacterium vaccae Increases Total Sleep and REM Sleep, and Changes NREM Architecture in Mice." *Sleep* 40, suppl. 1 (April 28, 2017): A55–A55. http://doi.org/10.1093/sleepj/zsx050.145.

Liu, Jiaming, Jing Sun, Fangyan Wang, Xichong Yu, Zongxin Ling, Haixiao Li, and Huiqing Zhang, et al. "Neuroprotective Effects of *Clostridium butyricum* against Vascular Dementia in Mice via Metabolic Butyrate." *BioMed Research International* 2015 (2015): 412946. http://doi.org/10.1155/2015/412946.

Mahnert, Alexander, Christine Moissl-Eichinger, and Gabriele Berg. "Microbiome Interplay: Plants Alter Microbial Abundance and Diversity Within the Built Environment." *Frontiers in Microbiology* 6, no. 491 (August 28, 2015): 887. http://doi.org/10.3389/fmicb.2015.00887.

Matthews, Dorothy M., and Susan M. Jenks. "Ingestion of *Mycobacterium vaccae* Decreases Anxiety-Related Behavior and Improves Learning in Mice." *Behavioural Processes* 96 (June 2013): 27–35. http://doi.org/10.1016/j.beproc.2013.02.007.

O'Brien, Mary E. R., H. Anderson, E. Kaukel, K. O'Byrne, M. Pawlicki, J. von Pawel, and M. Reck. "O-109 Improved Quality of Life with the Addition of SRL172 (Killed Mycobacterium vaccae) to Standard Chemotherapy in Patients with Advanced Non-Small Cell Lung Cancer: Phase III Results." *Lung Cancer* 41, suppl. 2 (August 2003): S35. http://doi.org/10.1016/S0169-5002(03)91767-3.

O'Brien, M. E. R., H. Anderson, E. Kaukel, K. O'Byrne, M. Pawlicki, J. Von Pawel, et al. "SRL172 (Killed Mycobacterium vaccae) in Addition to Standard Chemotherapy Improves Quality of Life Without Affecting Survival, in Patients with Advanced Non-Small-Cell Lung Cancer: Phase III Results." *Annals of Oncology: Official Journal of the European Society for Medical Oncology* 15, no. 6 (2004): 906–914.

Ramirez, Kelly S., Jonathan W. Leff, Albert Barberán, Scott Thomas Bates, Jason Betley, Thomas W. Crowther, and Eugene F. Kelly, et al. "Biogeographic Patterns in Below-Ground Diversity in New York City's Central Park Are Similar to Those Observed Globally." *Proceedings of the Royal Society B* 281, no. 1795 (October 1, 2014): 20141988. http://doi.org/10.1098/rspb.2014.1988.

Rebera, Stefan O., Philip H. Siebler, Nina C. Donner, James T. Morton, David G. Smith, Jared M. Kopelman, and Kenneth R. Lowe, et al. "Immunization with a Heat-Killed Preparation of the Environmental Bacterium *Mycobacterium vaccae* Promotes Stress Resilience in Mice." *Proceedings of the National Academy of Sciences of the United States of America* 113, no. 22 (May 31, 2016): E3130–9. http://doi.org/10.1073/pnas.1600324113.

Rook, Graham A. W., Christopher A. Lowry, and Charles L. Raison. "Microbial 'Old Friends,' Immunoregulation and Stress Resilience." *Evolution, Medicine, and Public Health* 2013, no. 1 (January 1, 2013): 46–64. http://doi.org/10.1093/emph/eot004.

Rook, Graham A. W., Charles L. Raison, and Christopher A. Lowry. "Can We Vaccinate Against Depression?" *Drug Discovery Today* 17, no. 9–10 (May 2012): 451–458. http://doi.org/10.1016/j.drudis.2012.03.018.

April: The Stardust in Us

American Psychological Association. *Stress in America: Our Health at Risk.* APA: January 11, 2012.

Bardgett, Mark E., Patrick J. Schultheis, Diana L. McGill, Raymond E. Richmond, and Jordan R. Wagge. "Magnesium Deficiency Impairs Fear Conditioning in Mice." *Brain Research* 1038, no. 1 (March 15, 2005): 100–106. http://doi.org/10.1016/j.brainres.2005.01.020.

El Baza, Farida, Heba Ahmed AlShahawi, Sally Zahra, and Rana Ahmed Abdel-Hakim. "Magnesium Supplementation in Children with Attention Deficit Hyperactivity Disorder." *Egyptian Journal of Medical Human Genetics* 17, no. 1 (January 2016): 63–70. http://doi.org/10.1016/j.ejmhg.2015.05.008.

Davis, D. R. "Declining Fruit and Vegetable Nutrient Composition: What Is the Evidence?" *HortScience* 44, no. 1 (February 2009): 15–19. http://hortsci.ashspublications.org/content/44/1/15.full.

Davis, Donald R. "Impact of Breeding and Yield on Fruit, Vegetable, and Grain Nutrient Content." In *Breeding for Fruit Quality*, edited by M. A. Jenks and P. J. Bebeli, 127–150. Hoboken, NJ: John Wiley & Sons, 2011. http://doi.org/10.1002/9780470959350.ch6.

Młynie, Katarzyna, Claire Linzi Davies, Irene Gómezde Agüero Sánchez, Karolina Pytka, Bogusława Budziszewska, and Gabriel Nowak. "Essential Elements in Depression and Anxiety. Part I." *Pharmacological Reports* 66, no. 4 (August 2014): 534–544. http://doi.org/10.1016/j.pharep.2014.03.001.

Montgomery, David R., and Anne Biklé. *The Hidden Half of Nature: The Microbial Roots of Life and Health.* New York: W. W. Norton, 2015.

Nalepa, Beata, Ewa Siemianowska, and Krystyna A. Skibniewska. "Influence of *Bifidobacterium bifidum* on Release of Minerals from Bread with Differing Bran Content." *Journal of Toxicology and Environmental Health, Part A* 75, no. 1 (November 2, 2011): 1–5. http://doi.org/10.1080/15287394.2011.615106.

Nielsen, Forrest H. "Relation between Magnesium Deficiency and Sleep Disorders and Associated Pathological Changes." In *Modulation of Sleep by Obesity, Diabetes, Age, and Diet*, edited by Ronald Ross Watson, 291–296. London: Academic Press, 2015. http://doi.org/10.1016/B978-0-12-420168-2.00031-4.

Nielsen, F. H., L. K. Johnson, and H. Zeng. "Magnesium Supplementation Improves Indicators of Low Magnesium Status and Inflammatory Stress in Adults Older than 51 Years with Poor Quality Sleep." *Magnesium Research* 23, no. 4 (December 2010): 158–168. http://doi.org/10.1684/mrh.2010.0220.

Pachikian, Barbara D., Audrey M. Neyrinck, Louise Deldicque, Fabienne C. De Backer, Emilie Catry, Evelyne M. Dewulf, and Florence M. Sohet, et al. "Changes in Intestinal Bifidobacteria Levels Are Associated with the Inflammatory Response in Magnesium-Deficient Mice." *Journal of Nutrition* 140, no. 3 (January 20, 2010): 509–514. http://doi.org/10.3945/jn.109.117374.

Sartori, S. B., N. Whittle, A. Hetzenauer, and N. Singewald. "Magnesium Deficiency Induces Anxiety and HPA Axis Dysregulation: Modulation by Therapeutic Drug Treatment." *Neuropharmacology* 62, no. 1 (January 2012): 304–312. http://doi.org/10.1016/j.neuropharm.2011.07.027.

van Ooijen, Gerben, and John S. O'Neill. "Intracellular Magnesium and the Rhythms of Life." *Cell Cycle* 15, no. 22 (July 27, 2016): 2997–2998. http://doi.org/10.1080/15384101.2016.1214030.

Watkins, K., and P. D. Josling. "A Pilot Study to Determine the Impact of Transdermal Magnesium Treatment on Serum Levels and Whole Body CaMg Ratios." *Nutrition Practitioner* (Spring 2010).

May: Can Green Help Gray Matter?

Aspinall, Peter, Panagiotis Mavros, Richard Coyne, and Jenny Roe. "The Urban Brain: Analysing Outdoor Physical Activity with Mobile EEG." *British Journal of Sports Medicine* 49, no. 4 (February 1, 2015): 272–276. http://doi.org/10.1136/bjsports-2012-091877.

Baird, Benjamin, Jonathan Smallwood, Michael D. Mrazek, Julia W. Y. Kam, Michael S. Franklin, and Jonathan W. Schooler. "Inspired by Distraction." *Psychological Science* 23, no. 10 (August 31, 2012): 1117–1122. http://doi.org/10.1177/0956797612446024.

Berman, Marc G., John Jonides, and Stephen Kaplan. "The Cognitive Benefits of Interacting with Nature." *Psychological Science* 19, no. 12 (December 1, 2008): 1207–1212. http://doi.org/10.1111/j.1467-9280.2008.02225.x.

Immordino-Yang, Mary Helen, Joanna A. Christodoulou, and Vanessa Singh. "Rest Is Not Idleness." *Perspectives on Psychological Science* 7, no. 4 (July 1, 2012): 352–364. http://doi.org/10.1177/1745691612447308.

Killingsworth, Matthew A., and Daniel T. Gilbert. "A Wandering Mind Is an Unhappy Mind." *Science* 330, no. 6006 (November 12, 2010): 932–932. http://doi.org/10.1126/science.1192439.

Kuo, Frances E., and Andrea Faber Taylor. "A Potential Natural Treatment for Attention-Deficit/Hyperactivity Disorder: Evidence from a National Study." *American Journal of Public Health* 94, no. 9 (September 1, 2004): 1580–1586. http://doi.org/10.2105/AJPH.94.9.1580.

Li, Dongying, and William C. Sullivan. "Impact of Views to School Landscapes on Recovery from Stress and Mental Fatigue." *Landscape and Urban Planning* 148 (April 2016): 149–158. http://doi.org/10.1016/j.landurbplan.2015.12.015.

Satish, Usha, Mark J. Mendell, Krishnamurthy Shekhar, Toshifumi Hotchi, Douglas Sullivan, Siegfried Streufert, and William J. Fisk. "Is CO_2 an Indoor Pollutant? Direct Effects of Low-to-Moderate CO_2 Concentrations on Human Decision-Making Performance." *Environmental Health Perspectives* 120, no. 2 (December 2012): 1671–7. http://doi.org/10.1289/ehp.1104789.

Smallwood, Jonathan, and Jessica Andrews-Hanna. "Not All Minds That Wander Are Lost: The Importance of a Balanced Perspective on the Mind-Wandering State." *Frontiers in Psychology* 4 (August 16, 2013): 441. http://doi.org/10.3389/fpsyg.2013.00441.

Taylor, Andrea Faber, and Frances E. Kuo. "Children with Attention Deficits Concentrate Better After Walk in the Park." *Journal of Attention Disorders* 12, no. 5 (March 1, 2009): 402–409. http://doi.org/10.1177/1087054708323000.

Taylor, Andrea Faber, Frances E. Kuo, andWilliam C. Sullivan. "Views of Nature and Self-Discipline: Evidence from Inner City Children." *Journal of Environmental Psychology* 22, no. 1–2 (March 2002): 49–63. http://doi.org/10.1006/jevp.2001.0241.

Valtchanov, Deltcho, Kevin R. Barton, and Colin Ellard. "Restorative Effects of Virtual Nature Settings." *Cyberpsychology, Behavior, and Social Networking* 13, no. 5 (October 17, 2010): 503–512. http://doi.org/10.1089/cyber.2009.0308.

Valtchanov, Deltcho, and Colin G. Ellard. "Cognitive and Affective Responses to Natural Scenes: Effects of Low Level Visual Properties on Preference, Cognitive Load and Eye-Movements." *Journal of Environmental Psychology* 43 (September 2015): 184–195. http://doi.org/10.1016/j.jenvp.2015.07.001.

June: Eternal Springtime of the Flavonoid Mind

Bell, Lynne, Daniel J. Lamport, Laurie T. Butler, and Claire M. Williams. "A Review of the Cognitive Effects Observed in Humans Following Acute Supplementation with Flavonoids, and Their Associated Mechanisms of Action." *Nutrients* 7, no. 12 (December 9, 2015): 10290–10306. http://doi.org/10.3390/nu7125538.

Beracochea, Daniel, Ali Krazem, Nadia Henkouss, Guillaume Haccard, Marc Roller, and Emilie Fromentin. "Intake of Wild Blueberry Powder Improves Episodic-Like and Working Memory during Normal Aging in Mice." *Planta Medica* 82, no. 13 (April 19, 2016): 1163–1168. http://doi.org/10.1055/s-0042-104419.

Brownmiller, Cindi, Luke R. Howard, and Ronald L. Prior. "Processing and Storage Effects on Procyanidin Composition and Concentration of Processed Blueberry Products." *Journal of Agricultural and Food Chemistry* 57, no. 5 (February 12, 2009): 1896–1902. http://doi.org/10.1021/jf803015s.

Del Bo', Cristian, Patrizia Riso, Ada Brambilla, Claudio Gardana, Anna Rizzolo, Paolo Simonetti, Gianni Bertolo, Dorothy Klimis-Zacas, and Marisa Porrini. "Blanching Improves Anthocyanin Absorption from Highbush Blueberry (*Vaccinium corymbosum* L.) Purée in Healthy Human Volunteers: A Pilot Study." *Journal of Agricultural and Food Chemistry* 60, no. 36 (August 20, 2012): 9298–9304. http://doi.org/10.1021/jf3021333.

Khalid, Sundus, Katie L. Barfoot, Gabrielle May, Daniel J. Lamport, Shirley A. Reynolds, and Claire M. Williams. "Effects of Acute Blueberry Flavonoids on Mood in Children and Young Adults." *Nutrients* 9, no. 2 (February 20, 2017): 158. http://doi.org/10.3390/nu9020158.

Krikorian, Robert, Marcelle D. Shidler, Tiffany A. Nash, Wilhelmina Kalt, Melinda R. Vinqvist-Tymchuk, Barbara Shukitt-Hale, and James A. Joseph. "Blueberry Supplementation Improves Memory in Older Adults." *Journal of Agricultural and Food Chemistry* 58, no. 7 (January 4, 2010): 3996–4000. http://doi.org/10.1021/jf9029332.

Lila, Mary Ann. "Anthocyanins and Human Health: An In Vitro Investigative Approach." *Journal of Biomedicine and Biotechnology* 2004, no. 5 (2004): 306–313. http://doi.org/10.1155/S111072430440401X.

Vendrame, Stefano, Simone Guglielmetti, Patrizia Riso, Stefania Arioli, Dorothy Klimis-Zacas, and Marisa Porrini. "Six-Week Consumption of a Wild Blueberry Powder Drink Increases Bifidobacteria in the Human Gut." *Journal of Agricultural and Food Chemistry* 59, no. 24 (November 7, 2011): 12815–12820. http://doi.org/10.1021/jf2028686.

Whyte, Adrian R., Graham Schafer, and Claire M. Williams. "Cognitive Effects Following Acute Wild Blueberry Supplementation in 7- to 10-Year-Old Children." *European Journal of Nutrition* 55, no. 6 (September 2016): 2151–2162. http://doi.org/10.1007/s00394-015-1029-4.

Whyte, Adrian R., and Claire M. Williams. "Effects of a Single Dose of a Flavonoid-Rich Blueberry Drink on Memory in 8 to 10 Y Old Children." *Nutrition* 31, no. 3 (March 2015): 531–534. http://doi.org/10.1016/j.nut.2014.09.013.

July: Uneven Playing Fields

Alloway, Ross G., and Tracy Packiam Alloway. "The Working Memory Benefits of Proprioceptively Demanding Training: A Pilot Study." *Perceptual and Motor Skills* 120, no. 3 (June 1, 2015): 766–775. http://doi.org/10.2466/22.PMS.120v18x1.

Alloway, Ross G., Tracy Packiam Alloway, Peter M. Magyari, and Shelley Floyd. "An Exploratory Study Investigating the Effects of Barefoot Running on Working Memory." *Perceptual and Motor Skills* 122, no. 2 (May 9, 2016): 432–443. http://doi.org/10.1177/0031512516640391.

Alloway, Tracy Packiam, and Ross G. Alloway. "Investigating the Predictive Roles of Working Memory and IQ in Academic Attainment." *Journal of Experimental Child Psychology* 106, no. 1 (May 2010): 20–29. http://doi.org/10.1016/j.jecp.2009.11.003.

Alloway, Tracy Packiam, and John C. Horton. "Does Working Memory Mediate the Link Between Dispositional Optimism and Depressive Symptoms?" *Applied Cognitive Psychology* 30, no. 6 (November/December 2016): 1068–1072. http://doi.org/10.1002/acp.3272.

Alloway, Tracy Packiam, Susan E. Gathercole, Catherine Willis, and Anne-Marie Adams. "A Structural Analysis of Working Memory and Related Cognitive Skills in Young Children." *Journal of Experimental Child Psychology* 87, no. 2 (February 2004): 85–106. http://doi.org/10.1016/j.jecp.2003.10.002.

Alloway, Tracy Packiam, and Maria Chiara Passolunghi. "The Relationship Between Working Memory, IQ, and Mathematical Skills in Children." *Learning and Individual Differences* 21, no. 1 (February 2011): 133–137. http://doi.org/10.1016/j.lindif.2010.09.013.

Alves, Christiano R. R., Victor H. Tessaro, Luis A. C. Teixeira, Karina Murakava, Hamilton Roschel, Bruno Gualano, and Monica Y. Takito. "Influence of Acute High-Intensity Aerobic Interval Exercise Bout on Selective Attention and Short-Term Memory Tasks." *Perceptual and Motor Skills* 118, no. 1 (February 1, 2014): 63–72. http://doi.org/10.2466/22.06.PMS.118k10w4.

Dehn, Milton J. *Working Memory and Academic Learning: Assessment and Intervention*. Hoboken, NJ: John Wiley & Sons, 2011.

Hale, James B., Jo-Ann B. Hoeppner, and Catherine A. Fiorello. "Analyzing Digit Span Components for Assessment of Attention Processes." *Journal of Psychoeducational Assessment* 20, no. 2 (June 1, 2002): 128–143. http://doi.org/10.1177/073428290202000202.

Hayter, A. L., D. W. Langdon, and N. Ramnani. "Cerebellar Contributions to Working Memory." *NeuroImage* 36, no. 3 (July 2007): 943–954. http://doi.org/10.1016/j.neuroimage.2007.03.011.

Koziol, Leonard F., Deborah Budding, Nancy Andreasen, Stefano D'Arrigo, Sara Bulgheroni, Hiroshi Imamizu, and Masao Ito, et al. "Consensus Paper: The Cerebellum's Role in Movement and Cognition." *Cerebellum* 13, no. 1 (February 2014): 151–177. http://doi.org/10.1007/s12311-013-0511-x.

Marvel, Cherie L., and John E. Desmond. "Functional Topography of the Cerebellum in Verbal Working Memory." *Neuropsychology Review* 20, no. 3 (September 2010): 271–279. http://doi.org/10.1007/s11065-010-9137-7.

Marvel, Cherie L., and John E. Desmond. "The Contributions of Cerebro-Cerebellar Circuitry to Executive Verbal Working Memory." *Cortex* 46, no. 7 (July–August 2010): 880–895. http://doi.org/10.1016/j.cortex.2009.08.017.

Roman, Adrienne S., David B. Pisoni, and William G. Kronenberger. "Assessment of Working Memory Capacity in Preschool Children Using the Missing Scan Task." *Infant and Child Development* 23, no. 6 (November/December 2014): 575–587. http://doi.org/10.1002/icd.1849.

Schmahmann, Jeremy D., and David Caplan. "Cognition, Emotion and the Cerebellum." *Brain* 129, no. 2 (February 2006): 290–292. https://doi.org/10.1093/brain/awh729.

Vandervert, Larry R., Paul H. Schimpf, and Hesheng Liu. "How Working Memory and the Cerebellum Collaborate to Produce Creativity and Innovation." *Creativity Research Journal* 19, no. 1 (December 5, 2007): 1–18. http://doi.org/10.1080/10400410709336873.

Weiss, Lawrence G., Donald H. Saklofske, Aurelio Prifitera, and James A. Hold-
nack. *WISC-IV Advanced Clinical Interpretation*. Cambridge, MA: Academic
Press, 2006.

August: The Right Touch

Benoit, Diane. "Infant-Parent Attachment: Definition, Types, Antecedents, Measurement and Outcome." *Paediatrics & Child Health* 9, no. 8 (2004): 541–545.
www.ncbi.nlm.nih.gov/pmc/articles/PMC2724160.

Brauer, Jens, Yaqiong Xiao, Tanja Poulain, Angela D. Friederici, and Annett
Schirmer. "Frequency of Maternal Touch Predicts Resting Activity and Connectivity of the Developing Social Brain." *Cerebral Cortex* 26, no. 8 (August 2016): 3544–3552. http://doi.org/10.1093/cercor/bhw137.

Coan, James A., Hillary S. Schaefer, and Richard J. Davidson. "Lending a Hand:
Social Regulation of the Neural Response to Threat." *Psychological Science*
17, no. 12 (December 1, 2016): 1032–1039. http://doi.org/10.1111/j.1467
-9280.2006.01832.x.

Guéguen, Nicolas. "Nonverbal Encouragement of Participation in a Course: The
Effect of Touching." *Social Psychology of Education* 7, no. 1 (March 2004):
89–98. https://doi.org/10.1023/B:SPOE.0000010691.30834.14.

Guéguen, Nicolas, and Jacques Fischer-Lokou. "An Evaluation of Touch on a
Large Request: A Field Setting." *Psychological Reports* 90, no. 1 (Feburary 1,
2002): 267–269. http://doi.org/10.2466/pr0.2002.90.1.267.

Hertenstein, Matthew J., Rachel Holmes, Margaret McCullough, and Dacher
Keltner. "The Communication of Emotion via Touch." *Emotion* 9, no. 4 (August 2009): 566–573. http://doi.org/10.1037/a0016108.

Hertenstein, Matthew J., and Dacher Keltner. "Gender and the Communication of
Emotion Via Touch." *Sex Roles* 64, no. 1–2 (January 2011): 70–80. http://doi
.org/10.1007/s11199-010-9842-y.

Hertenstein, Matthew J., and Sandra J. Weiss. *The Handbook of Touch: Neuroscience, Behavioral, and Health Perspectives*. New York: Springer, 2011.

Leonard, Julia A., Talia Berkowitz, and Anna Shusterman. "The Effect of Friendly
Touch on Delay-of-Gratification in Preschool Children." *Quarterly Journal of
Experimental Psychology* 67, no. 11 (2014): 2123–2133. http://doi.org/10.1080
/17470218.2014.907325.

Linden, David J. *Touch: The Science of the Hand, Heart, and Mind*. New York:
Penguin, 2015.

Oveis, Christopher, June Gruber, Dacher Keltner, Juliet L. Stamper, and W. Thomas Boyce. "Smile Intensity and Warm Touch as Thin Slices of Child and Family Affective Style." *Emotion* 9, no. 4 (August 2009): 544–548. http://doi.org/10.1037/a0016300.

Patterson, Miles L., Jack L. Powell, and Mary G. Lenihan. "Touch, Compliance, and Interpersonal Affect." *Journal of Nonverbal Behavior* 10, no. 1 (March 1986): 41–50. http://doi.org/10.1007/BF00987204.

Sharp, Helen, Andrew Pickles, Michael Meaney, Kate Marshall, Florin Tibu, and Jonathan Hill. "Frequency of Infant Stroking Reported by Mothers Moderates the Effect of Prenatal Depression on Infant Behavioural and Physiological Outcomes." *PloS One* 7, no. 10 (October 16, 2012): e45446. http://doi.org/10.1371/journal.pone.0045446.

Weaver, Ian C. G. "Epigenetic Programming by Maternal Behavior and Pharmacological Intervention *Nature Versus Nurture: Let's Call The Whole Thing Off.*" *Epigenetics* 2, no. 1 (2007): 22–28. http://doi.org/10.4161/epi.2.1.3881.

September: 99 Percent Perspiration

Brooks, Alison W. "Get Excited: Reappraising Pre-Performance Anxiety as Excitement." *Journal of Experimental Psychology: General* 143, no. 3 (June 2014): 1144–1158. http://doi.org/10.1037/a0035325.

Chen, Denise, Ameeta Katdare, and Nadia Lucas. "Chemosignals of Fear Enhance Cognitive Performance in Humans." *Chemical Senses* 31, no. 5 (June 2006): 415–423. https://doi.org/10.1093/chemse/bjj046.

Dalton, Pamela, Christopher Mauté, Cristina Jaén, and Tamika Wilson. "Chemosignals of Stress Influence Social Judgments." *PloS One* 8, no. 10 (October 9, 2013): e77144. http://doi.org/10.1371/journal.pone.0077144.

de Groot, Jasper H. B., Monique A. M. Smeets, Annemarie Kaldewaij, Maarten J. A. Duijndam, and Gün R. Semin. "Chemosignals Communicate Human Emotions." *Psychological Science* 23, no. 11 (November 2012): 1417–1424. http://doi.org/10.1177/0956797612445317.

Doty, Richard L. *Handbook of Olfaction and Gustation.* Hoboken, NJ: John Wiley & Sons, 2015.

Dougherty, Lea R., Sarah L. Blankenship, Philip A. Spechler, Srikanth Padmala, and Luiz Pessoa. "An fMRI Pilot Study of Cognitive Reappraisal in Children: Divergent Effects on Brain and Behavior." *Journal of Psychopathology*

and Behavioral Assessment 37, no. 4 (December 2015): 634–644. http://doi
.org/10.1007/s10862-015-9492-z.

Jamieson, Jeremy P., Wendy Berry Mendes, Erin Blackstock, and Toni Schmad-
er. "Turning the Knots in Your Stomach into Bows: Reappraising Arousal
Improves Performance on the GRE." *Journal of Experimental Social Psychology* 46, no. 1 (January 2010): 208–212. http://doi.org/10.1016/j.jesp.2009
.08.015.

Lübke, Katrin T., Anne Busch, Matthias Hoenen, Benoist Schaal, and Bettina
M. Pause. "Chemosensory Anxiety Signals Prime Defensive Behavior in
Prepubertal Girls." *Physiology & Behavior* 173 (May 2017): 30–33. http://doi
.org/10.1016/j.physbeh.2017.01.035.

Lübke, Katrin T., and Bettina M. Pause. "Always Follow Your Nose: The Functional Significance of Social Chemosignals in Human Reproduction and
Survival." *Hormones and Behavior* 68 (February 2015): 134–144. http://doi
.org/10.1016/j.yhbeh.2014.10.001.

Parma, Valentina, Amy R. Gordon, Cinzia Cecchetto, Annachiara Cavazzana,
Johan N. Lundström, and Mats J. Olsson. "Processing of Human Body
Odors." In *Springer Handbook of Odor*, 3rd ed., Vol. 123, edited by Andrea
Buettner, 127–128. New York: Springer, 2017. http://doi.org/10.1007/978-3
-319-26932-0_51.

Pause, Bettina M. "Processing of Body Odor Signals by the Human Brain." *Chemosensory Perception* 5, no. 1 (March 2012): 55–63. http://doi.org/10.1007
/s12078-011-9108-2.

Pincott, Jena. *Do Gentlemen Really Prefer Blondes? Bodies, Behavior, and Brains—
The Science Behind Sex, Love, & Attraction*. New York: Delta, 2009.

Prehn, Alexander, Anne Ohrt, Bernfried Sojka, Roman Ferstl, and Bettina
M. Pause. "Chemosensory Anxiety Signals Augment the Startle Reflex in
Humans." *Neuroscience Letters* 394, no. 2 (February 2006): 127–130. http://
doi.org/10.1016/j.neulet.2005.10.012.

Rubin, Denis, Yevgeny Botanov, Greg Hajcak, and Lilianne R. Mujica-Parodi.
"Second-Hand Stress: Inhalation of Stress Sweat Enhances Neural Response
to Neutral Faces." *Social Cognitive and Affective Neuroscience* 7, no. 2 (February 2012): 208–212. https://doi.org/10.1093/scan/nsq097.

Zhou, Wen, and Denise Chen. "Fear-Related Chemosignals Modulate Recogni-
tion of Fear in Ambiguous Facial Expressions." *Psychological Science* 20, no. 2
(February 2009): 177–183. http://doi.org/10.1111/j.1467-9280.2009.02263.x.

Zhou, Wen, and Denise Chen. "Sociochemosensory and Emotional Functions." *Psychological Science* 20, no. 9 (September 2009): 1118–1124. http://doi .org/10.1111/j.1467-9280.2009.02413.x.

October: City Brain

Abbott, Alison. "City Living Marks the Brain." *Nature* 474, no. 7352 (June 23, 2011): 429. http://doi.org/10.1038/474429a.

Baikie, Karen A., and Kay Wilhelm. "Emotional and Physical Health Benefits of Expressive Writing." *Advances in Psychiatric Treatment* 11, no. 5 (August 2005): 338–346. http://doi.org/10.1192/apt.11.5.338.

Giannotta, Fabrizia, Michele Settanni, Wendy Kliewer, and Silvia Ciairano. "Results of an Italian School-Based Expressive Writing Intervention Trial Focused on Peer Problems." *Journal of Adolescence* 32, no. 6 (December 2009): 1377–1389. http://doi.org/10.1016/j.adolescence.2009.07.001.

Golembiewski, Jan A. "The Designed Environment and How It Affects Brain Morphology and Mental Health." *HERD: Health Environments Research & Design Journal* 9, no. 2 (November 23, 2015): 161–171. http://doi .org/10.1177/1937586715609562.

Holz, Nathalie E., Manfred Laucht, and Andreas Meyer-Lindenberg. "Recent Advances in Understanding the Neurobiology of Childhood Socioeconomic Disadvantage." *Current Opinion in Psychiatry* 28, no. 5 (September 2015): 365–370. http://doi.org/10.1097/YCO.0000000000000178.

Kliewer, Wendy, Stephen J. Lepore, Albert D. Farrell, Kevin W. Allison, Aleta L. Meyer, Terri N. Sullivan, and Anne Y. Greene. "A School-Based Expressive Writing Intervention for At-Risk Urban Adolescents' Aggressive Behavior and Emotional Lability." *Journal of Clinical Child & Adolescent Psychology* 40, no. 5 (September 14, 2011): 693–705. http://doi.org/10.1080/15374416 .2011.597092.

Le Hunte, Bem, and Jan A. Golembiewski. "Stories Have the Power to Save Us: A Neurological Framework for the Imperative to Tell Stories." *Arts and Social Sciences Journal* 5, no. 73 (July 28, 2014). http://doi.org/10.4172 /2151-6200.1000073.

Lederbogen, Florian, Peter Kirsch, Leila Haddad, Fabian Streit, Heike Tost, Philipp Schuch, and Stefan Wüst, et al. "City Living and Urban Upbringing Affect Neural Social Stress Processing in Humans." *Nature* 474, no. 7352 (June 23, 2011): 498–501. http://doi.org/10.1038/nature10190.

Lieberman, Matthew D., Naomi I. Eisenberger, Molly J. Crockett, Sabrina M. Tom, Jennifer H. Pfeifer, and Baldwin M. Way. "Putting Feelings Into Words." *Psychological Science* 18, no. 5 (May 1, 2007): 421–428. http://doi .org/10.1111/j.1467-9280.2007.01916.x.

Meyer-Lindenberg, Andreas. "Big City Blues." *Scientific American Mind* 24, no. 1 (March/April 2013): 58–61. https://doi.org/10/1038/scientificamerican mind0313-58.

Niles, Andrea N., Kate E. Byrne Haltom, Matthew D. Lieberman, Christopher Hur, and Annette L. Stanton. "Writing Content Predicts Benefit from Written Expressive Disclosure: Evidence for Repeated Exposure and Self-Affirmation." *Cognition & Emotion* 30, no. 2 (2016): 258–274. http://doi.org/10.1080/0269 9931.2014.995598.

Pennebaker, James W., and Janel D. Seagal. "Forming a Story: The Health Benefits of Narrative." *Journal of Clinical Psychology* 55, no. 10 (September 30, 1999): 1243–1254. http://doi.org/10.1002/(SICI)1097-4679(199910)55:10<1243::AID -JCLP6>3.0.CO;2-N.

Ramirez, Gerardo, and Sian L. Beilock. "Writing About Testing Worries Boosts Exam Performance in the Classroom." *Science* 331, no. 6014 (January 14, 2011): 211–213. http://doi.org/10.1126/science.1199427.

Spencer, C., and H. Woolley. "Children and the City: A Summary of Recent Environmental Psychology Research." *Child: Care, Health and Development* 26, no. 3 (May 2000): 181–198. http://doi.org/10.1046/j.1365-2214.2000.00125.x.

Tabibnia, Golnaz, Matthew D. Lieberman, and Michelle G. Craske. "The Lasting Effect of Words on Feelings: Words May Facilitate Exposure Effects to Threatening Images." *Emotion* 8, no. 3 (June 2008): 307–317. http://doi.org/10 .1037/1528-3542.8.3.307.

Takooshian, Harold, S. Haber, and D. J. Lucido. "Who Wouldnt Help a Lost Child? You, Maybe." *Psychology Today*, February 1977, 67–68, 88.

November: Rage Against the Dying of the Light

Abdullah, Saeed, Mary Czerwinski, Gloria Mark, and Paul Johns. "Shining (Blue) Light on Creative Ability." In *Proceedings of the 2016 ACM International Joint Conference on Pervasive and Ubiquitous Computing*, edited by Ubi-Comp 2016, 793–804. New York: ACM, September 12–16, 2016. http://doi .org/10.1145/2971648.2971751.

Burgess, Helen J., and Thomas A. Molina. "Home Lighting Before Usual Bedtime Impacts Circadian Timing: A Field Study." *Photochemistry and Photobiology* 90, no. 3 (February 7, 2014): 723–726. http://doi.org/10.1111/php.12241.

Cavallo, Anita. "Melatonin and Human Puberty: Current Perspectives." *Journal of Pineal Research* 15, no. 3 (October 1993): 115–121. http://doi.org/10.1111/j.1600-079X.1993.tb00517.x.

Choi, Kyungah, and Hyeon-Jeong Suk. "Dynamic Lighting System for the Learning Environment: Performance of Elementary Students." *Optics Express* 24, no. 10 (2016): A907–16. http://doi.org/10.1364/OE.24.00A907.

Correa, Ángel, Antonio Barba, and Francisca Padilla. "Light Effects on Behavioural Performance Depend on the Individual State of Vigilance." *PloS One* 11, no. 11 (November 7, 2016): e0164945. http://doi.org/10.1371/journal.pone.0164945.

Crowley, Stephanie J., Sean W. Cain, Angus C. Burns, Christine Acebo, and Mary A. Carskadon. "Increased Sensitivity of the Circadian System to Light in Early/Mid-Puberty." *Journal of Clinical Endocrinology and Metabolism* 100, no. 11 (November 1, 2015): 4067–4073. http://doi.org/10.1210/jc.2015-2775.

Gabel, Virginie, Micheline Maire, Carolin F. Reichert, Sarah L. Chellappa, Christina Schmidt, Vanja Hommes, Antoine U. Viola, and Christian Cajochen. "Effects of Artificial Dawn and Morning Blue Light on Daytime Cognitive Performance, Well-Being, Cortisol and Melatonin Levels." *Chronobiology International* 30, no. 8 (2013): 988–997. http://doi.org/10.3109/07420528.2013.793196.

Higuchi, Shigekazu, Yuki Nagafuchi, Sang-il Lee, and Tetsuo Harada. "Influence of Light at Night on Melatonin Suppression in Children." *Journal of Clinical Endocrinology & Metabolism* 99, no. 9 (September 2014): 3298–3303. https://doi.org/10.1210/jc.2014-1629.

Kang, Seung-Gul, Ho-Kyoung Yoon, Chul-Hyun Cho, Soonwook Kwon, June Kang, Young-Min Park, Eunil Lee, Leen Kim, and Heon-Jeong Lee. "Decrease in fMRI Brain Activation During Working Memory Performed After Sleeping under 10 Lux Light." *Scientific Reports* 6, no. 36731 (November 6, 2016). http://doi.org/10.1038/srep36731.

Piekarski, David J., Josiah R. Boivin, and Linda Wilbrecht. "Ovarian Hormones Organize the Maturation of Inhibitory Neurotransmission in the Frontal Cortex at Puberty Onset in Female Mice." *Current Biology* 27, no. 12 (June 2017): 1735–1745.e3. http://doi.org/10.1016/j.cub.2017.05.027.

Reiter, Russel J., Dun-Xian Tan, Ahmet Korkmaz, Thomas C. Erren, Claus Piek-arski, Hiroshi Tamura, and Lucien C. Manchester. "Light at Night, Chronodisruption, Melatonin Suppression, and Cancer Risk: A Review." *Critical Reviews in Oncogenesis* 13, no. 4 (2007): 303–328. http://doi.org/10.1615/CritRevOncog.v13.i4.30.

Soares de Holanda, Felisbela, Sérgio Tufik, Magda Bignotto, Carla G. Maganhin, Lucia Helena Laprano Vieira, Edmund C. Baracat, and José Maria Soares Jr. "Evaluation of Melatonin on the Precocious Puberty: A Pilot Study." *Gynecological Endocrinology* 27, no. 8 (2011): 519–523. http://doi.org/10.3109/09513590.2010.501888.

Steidle, Anna, and Lioba Werth. "Freedom from Constraints: Darkness and Dim Illumination Promote Creativity." *Journal of Environmental Psychology* 35 (September 2013): 67–80. http://doi.org/10.1016/j.jenvp.2013.05.003.

Steingraber, Sandra. *The Falling Age of Puberty in US Girls: What We Know, What We Need to Know.* San Francisco: Breast Cancer Fund, 2007.

Tamura, Hiroshi, Yasuhiko Nakamura, Ahmet Korkmaz, Lucien C. Manchester, Dun-Xian Tan, Norihiro Sugino, and Russel J. Reiter. "Melatonin and the Ovary: Physiological and Pathophysiological Implications." *Fertility and Sterility* 92, no. 1 (July 2009): 328–343. http://doi.org/10.1016/j.fertnstert.2008.05.016.

Vartanian, Garen V., Benjamin Y. Li, Andrew P. Chervenak, Oliva J. Walch, Weston Pack, Petri Ala-Laurila, and Kwoon Y. Wong. "Melatonin Suppression by Light in Humans Is More Sensitive Than Previously Reported." *Journal of Biological Rhythms* 30, no. 4 (August 1, 2015): 351–354. http://doi.org/10.1177/0748730415585413.

West, Kathleen E., Michael R. Jablonski, Benjamin Warfield, Kate S. Cecil, Mary James, Melissa A. Ayers, and James Maida, et al. "Blue Light from Light-Emitting Diodes Elicits a Dose-Dependent Suppression of Melatonin in Humans." *Journal of Applied Physiology* 110, no. 3 (March 1, 2011): 619–626. http://doi.org/10.1152/japplphysiol.01413.2009.

Wright, Kenneth P., Jr., Andrew W. McHill, Brian R. Birks, Brandon R. Griffin, Thomas Rusterholz, and Evan D. Chinoy. "Entrainment of the Human Circadian Clock to the Natural Light-Dark Cycle." *Current Biology* 23, no. 16 (August 1, 2013): 1554–1558. http://doi.org/10.1016/j.cub.2013.06.039.

December: All Is Calm, All Is Bright

Appelhans, Bradley M., and Linda J. Luecken. "Heart Rate Variability as an Index of Regulated Emotional Responding." *Review of General Psychology* 10, no. 3 (September 2006): 229–240. http://doi.org/10.1037/1089-2680.10.3.229.

Bornemann, Boris, Bethany E. Kok, Anne Böckler, and Tania Singer. "Helping from the Heart: Voluntary Upregulation of Heart Rate Variability Predicts Altruistic Behavior." *Biological Psychology* 119 (September 2016): 54–63. http://doi.org/10.1016/j.biopsycho.2016.07.004.

Denson, Thomas F., Jessica R. Grisham, and Michelle L. Moulds. "Cognitive Reappraisal Increases Heart Rate Variability in Response to an Anger Provocation." *Motivation and Emotion* 35, no. 1 (March 2011): 14–22. http://doi.org/10.1007/s11031-011-9201-5.

DiPietro, Janet A., Marc H. Bornstein, Chun-Shin Hahn, Kathleen Costigan, and Aristide Achy-Brou. "Fetal Heart Rate and Variability: Stability and Prediction to Developmental Outcomes in Early Childhood." *Child Development* 78, no. 6 (November/December 2007): 1788–1798. http://doi.org/10.1111/j.1467-8624.2007.01099.x.

Draghici, Adina E., and J. Andrew Taylor. "The Physiological Basis and Measurement of Heart Rate Variability in Humans." *Journal of Physiological Anthropology* 35 (September 28, 2016): 22. http://doi.org/10.1186/s40101-016-0113-7.

Fenton-O'Creevy, Mark, Jeffrey T. Lins, Shalini Vohra, Daniel W. Richards, Gareth Davies, and Kristina Schaaff. "Emotion Regulation and Trader Expertise: Heart Rate Variability on the Trading Floor." *Journal of Neuroscience, Psychology, and Economics* 5, no. 4 (November 2012): 227–237. http://doi.org/10.1037/a0030364.

Gevirtz, Richard. "Integrating Heart Rate Variability Biofeedback into Mindfulness-Based Therapies." *Biofeedback* 43, no. 3 (Fall 2015): 129–132. http://doi.org/10.5298/1081-5937-43.3.03.

Gladwell, Valerie F., Pekka Kuoppa, Mika P. Tarvainen, and Mike Rogerson. "A Lunchtime Walk in Nature Enhances Restoration of Autonomic Control during Night-Time Sleep: Results from a Preliminary Study." *International Journal of Environmental Research and Public Health* 13, no. 3 (March 3, 2016): 280. http://doi.org/10.3390/ijerph13030280.

Grossmann, Igor, Baljinder K. Sahdra, and Joseph Ciarrochi. "A Heart and a Mind: Self-Distancing Facilitates the Association Between Heart Rate Variability, and Wise Reasoning." *Frontiers in Behavioral Neuroscience* 10 (April 8, 2016): 68. http://doi.org/10.3389/fnbeh.2016.00068.

Lagos, Leah, Evgeny Vaschillo, Bronya Vaschillo, Paul Lehrer, Marsha Bates, and Robert Pandina. "Virtual Reality–Assisted Heart Rate Variability Biofeedback as a Strategy to Improve Golf Performance: A Case Study." *Biofeedback* 39, no. 1 (Spring 2011): 15–20. http://doi.org/10.5298/1081-5937-39.1.11.

Massin, M., and G. von Bernuth. "Normal Ranges of Heart Rate Variability During Infancy and Childhood." *Pediatric Cardiology* 18, no. 4 (July 1997): 297–302. http://doi.org/10.1007/s002469900178.

Michels, Nathalie, Els Clays, Marc De Buyzere, Inge Huybrechts, Staffan Marild, Barbara Vanaelst, Stefaan De Henauw, and Isabelle Sioen. "Determinants and Reference Values of Short-Term Heart Rate Variability in Children." *European Journal of Applied Physiology* 113, no. 6 (June 2013): 1477–1488. http://doi.org/10.1007/s00421-012-2572-9.

Miller, Jonas G., Sarah Kahle, and Paul D. Hastings. "Roots and Benefits of Costly Giving." *Psychological Science* 26, no. 7 (May 26, 2015): 1038–1045. http://doi.org/10.1177/0956797615578476.

Ononogbu, Sandra, Marjut Wallenius, Raija-Leena Punamäki, Lea Saarni, Harri Lindholm, and Clas-Håkan Nygård. "Association between Information and Communication Technology Usage and the Quality of Sleep among School-Aged Children during a School Week." *Sleep Disorders* 2014 (January 28, 2014): 315808. http://doi.org/10.1155/2014/315808.

Park, Sung Kyun, Katherine L. Tucker, Marie S. O'Neill, David Sparrow, Pantel S. Vokonas, Howard Hu, and Joel Schwartz. "Fruit, Vegetable, and Fish Consumption and Heart Rate Variability: The Veterans Administration Normative Aging Study." *American Journal of Clinical Nutrition* 89, no. 3 (March 2009): 778–786. http://doi.org/10.3945/ajcn.2008.26849.

Perrotta, Andrew S., Andrew T. Jeklin, Ben A. Hives, Leah E. Meanwell, and Darren E. R. Warburton. "Validity of the Elite HRV Smartphone Application for Examining Heart Rate Variability in a Field-Based Setting." *Journal of Strength and Conditioning Research* 31, no. 8 (August 2017): 2296–2302. http://doi.org/10.1519/JSC.0000000000001841.

Plews, Daniel J., Ben Scott, Marco Altini, Matt Wood, Andrew E. Kilding, and Paul B. Laursen. "Comparison of Heart Rate Variability Recording with Smart Phone Photoplethysmographic, Polar H7 Chest Strap and Electrocardiogram

Methods." *International Journal of Sports Physiology and Performance* (n.d.): 1–17. http://doi.org/10.1123/ijspp.2016-0668.

Rennie, Kirsten L., Harry Hemingway, Meena Kumari, Eric Brunner, Marek Malik, and Michael Marmot. "Effects of Moderate and Vigorous Physical Activity on Heart Rate Variability in a British Study of Civil Servants." *American Journal of Epidemiology* 158, no. 2 (July 15, 2003): 135–143. https://doi.org/10.1093/aje/kwg120.

Sahdra, Baljinder K., Joseph Ciarrochi, and Philip D. Parker. "High-Frequency Heart Rate Variability Linked to Affiliation with a New Group." *PloS One* 10, no. 6 (June 24, 2015): e0129583. http://doi.org/10.1371/journal.pone.0129583.

Sammito, Stefan, and Irina Böckelmann. "New Reference Values of Heart Rate Variability During Ordinary Daily Activity." *Heart Rhythm* 14, no. 2 (February 2017): 304–307. http://doi.org/10.1016/j.hrthm.2016.12.016.

Seeley, Saren H., Betina Yanez, Annette L. Stanton, and Michael A. Hoyt. "An Emotional Processing Writing Intervention and Heart Rate Variability: The Role of Emotional Approach." *Cognition & Emotion* 31, no. 5 (April 15, 2016): 988–994. http://doi.org/10.1080/02699931.2016.1170667.

Sun, Lihua, Jari Peräkylä, Katri Holm, Joonas Haapasalo, Kai Lehtimäki, Keith H. Ogawa, Jukka Peltola, and Kaisa M. Hartikainen. "Vagus Nerve Stimulation Improves Working Memory Performance." *Journal of Clinical and Experimental Neuropsychology* 14, no. 1 (2017): 1–11. http://doi.org/10.1080/13803395.2017.1285869.

Index

About the Author

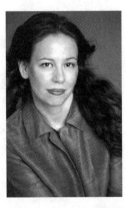

JENA PINCOTT IS the author of *Do Chocolate Lovers Have Sweeter Babies?*, which received starred reviews from *Library Journal* and *Kirkus* for mixing "science with wit, personal anecdote, and playful humor," and *Do Gentlemen Really Prefer Blondes?*, on the science of love and attraction, which received a starred review from *Publishers Weekly* and has been translated into eighteen languages. Her science writing and interviews have appeared in *Psychology Today*, the *Wall Street Journal*, *Nautilus*, the *Huffington Post*, *Brain World Magazine*, Oprah.com/OWN, and many other outlets. She lives with her husband and two daughters in New York City.